Enhancing Hospital Efficiency

The study described in this book was made possible by financial contributions from The Sergei S. Zlinkoff Fund for Medical Research and Education. Royalties from the sale of the book will go to The Valley Hospital Foundation.

The authors express thanks and personal gratitude to Mrs. Barbara Rooney whose participation and interest in the project made this book possible.

ENHANCING HOSPITAL EFFICIENCY

A Guide to
Expanding Beds without Bricks

A STUDY OF FIFTEEN HOSPITALS

JOHN PETERSON
DAVID MANCHESTER
ARTHUR TOAN

AUPHA Press
Washington, D.C. • Ann Arbor, Michigan

Library of Congress Cataloguing in Publication Data

Peterson, John, 1918–
    Enhancing hospital efficiency.

    Bibliography: p.
    Includes index.
    1. Hospitals — Administration. 2. Hospital utiliza-
tion. 3. Medical appointments and schedules.
4. Hospital care. 5. Hospital and community.
I. Manchester, David, joint author. II. Toan,
Arthur B., joint author. III. Title. [DNLM:
1. Hospital bed capacity. 2. Hospital administration.
3. Hospitals — Utilization. WX153 P485e]
RA971.P49   362.1'1'0685   80-15724
ISBN 0-914904-45-0
ISBN 0-914904-46-9 (pbk.)

AUPHA Press is an imprint of Health Administration Press.

Health Administration Press   AUPHA Press
School of Public Health   One DuPont Circle
University of Michigan   Washington, D.C. 20036
Ann Arbor, Michigan 48109   202–659–4354
313–764–1380

Foreword

In the 1980s the skills of hospital administrators must be increasingly devoted to improving the efficiency of the health care system as a whole. The most successful managers of the coming decade will be those who meet the widespread and growing consensus among our constituencies demanding that hospitals and doctors continue to provide first-class service without substantial increases in the cost burden. The health care industry must join many other sectors of society in improving overall productivity. Like automakers, educators, and government managers, we must learn to do more with limited resources. It is clear that no minor or temporary adjustments are sufficient. Rather, we must turn to fundamental reconsiderations of both the services we give and the ways we deliver them.

In that context, the authors of this book have made a unique and highly imaginative contribution. As part of the long-range planning process for The Valley Hospital of Ridgewood, New Jersey, John Peterson, a hospital executive with many years of experience, David Manchester, a young hospital administrator, and Arthur Toan, a hospital trustee and a retired partner of a major accounting firm, elected to visit 14 medium to large-sized voluntary community hospitals throughout the United States. The places they selected are exceptionally well-respected institutions. The questions they asked dealt basically with the hospital's ability to provide more service to its physicians and patients without expanding its present bed supply. The authors assumed, correctly and wisely, that hospitals and doctors collaborate to provide effective service, and that the collaboration extends both into the management of the hospital itself and into the practice of medicine.

Their report shows how, based on that collaboration, several leading institutions addressed a number of efficiency issues. These include ways in which hospitals can increase their occupancy, shorten their length of stay, and increase outpatient services, and ways they can assist physicians in their practice away from the hospital. Finally, the authors address issues of the hospital's roles in the prevention of disease and in effective interaction with other "publics." The authors conclude by considering another fundamental question: the role of the hospital in maintaining an appropriate number and variety of physicians for their communities.

This is a work by practitioners for practitioners. Unlike academic studies with rigorous documentation and quantification, the authors' report is a qualitative and conceptual review of the possibilities and the achievements of their own institution and the others they visited. Rigorous quantification of the broad range of ideas they discussed was well beyond their purposes or resources. Research groups, particularly the ones led by Dr. Walton M. Hancock, The University of Michigan, and Dr. Donald Holloway, the University of California at Berkeley and Alta Bates Hospital, have provided scholarly studies supporting many of the concepts now being applied in the 15 hospitals. Readers interested in these studies might refer to the bibliography.

John R. Griffith
Chairman
Editorial Board
Health Administration Press
Ann Arbor, Michigan
March, 1980

Contents

Chapter

  I. Introduction and Summary   1

  II. Making the Hospital an Efficient Instrument through
Policies and Practices Concerning Capacity, Scheduling,
Cancellations, and Discharges   11
    Maximizing the Availability of Beds during Periods
      of Peak Demand   12
    Off-peak Utilization   21
    Outpatient or One-day Surgery   26
    Scheduling, Admitting, and Cancelling   28
    Discharge Management   36

  III. Making the Hospital an Efficient Instrument through
Responsive Ancillary and Other Hospital-based Services   41
    Radiology Services   42
    Laboratory Services   51
    The Desirability of Providing Outpatient Services   58
    Preadmission Testing   59
    Operating Rooms   62
    Physical Therapy Services   71
    Patient Transport and Scheduling   71
    The Availability of Consultants   73

  IV. Facilitating the Efficient Use of the Hospital by
Attending Physicians   75
    Lengths of Stay in the Individual Hospital   76
    Variations in Lengths of Stay among Hospitals   82
    Length of Stay in Obstetrical Services   88
    Some General Comments on Physician Efficiency   90
    Medical Office Buildings   92

V. Making Appropriate Use of Alternatives to Hospital
Care: The Effective Use of Other Community Resources   95
The Hospital as Part of the Health Care System   95
Doctors as Part of the Health Care System   108

VI. Informing, Influencing, and Adapting to the Hospital's
Environment   111

VII. Census Control through Medical Staff Regulation
and Limitation   117

VIII. Conclusion   121

Appendixes
1. A Brief Description of The Valley Hospital   133
2. A Case Study: "Getting the Most Out of the Hospital"   134
Selected Bibliography   137
Index   139

Tables

III–1	In-House Radiologist Availability	44
III–2	Examples of Technical Staff Coverage — Radiology and Laboratory Departments	45
III–3	In-House Pathology Availability	46
III–4	OR Availability for Elective Cases	65
IV–1	Comparative Length of Stay (1978): Twelve Representative Diagnoses	83
V–1	Preventive Medicine and Public Education	98

I

Introduction and Summary

DESCRIPTION OF STUDY

ORIGIN AND OBJECTIVES OF STUDY

It comes as a surprise to many, at a time when major attention is being focused on the surplus of hospital beds, that a significant number of individual hospitals have problems of overcrowding. The Valley Hospital is one of these.*

Valley has operated successfully for many years on the premise that a low-length-of-stay, high-occupancy hospital, with a high level of activity and a participative medical staff, can provide a large volume of high quality care at a reasonable cost. It plans to continue to do so.

Its present problems arise from the fact that local and state regulatory restrictions prevent it from expanding to meet the demands being placed on it. More particularly, Valley is faced with:

1. A high occupancy rate — particularly in the medical/surgical area, where it exceeds 90 percent.
2. A continued, although slow, growth in patient admissions of about 2 percent a year.
3. Continued pressure by doctors for admission to a medical staff that now numbers 262 active staff physicians and 20 dentists.
4. An inability to expand either building or parking space in the face of zoning laws and the opposition of neighbors to the acquisition of surrounding homes.

---

* A brief description of The Valley Hospital is included as Appendix 1.

5. Decisions of the local Health Systems Agency (HSA) for Bergen and Passaic Counties and of the New Jersey Department of Health not to permit an increase in the number of beds in the HSA and state area.

The research project presented here grew out of our conviction that we could improve our ability to meet the demands being placed on the hospital by tapping the knowledge and experience of people in other institutions with similar conditions.

We recognized that no way exists by which Valley or any other hospital can indefinitely increase its ability to treat patients or to admit additional doctors to its medical staff. Nevertheless, there seemed to be enough value in trying to find ways to increase Valley's effective capacity, through raising the rate of occupancy and reducing the length of stay of patients, to warrant the efforts to do so.

NATURE AND SCOPE OF STUDY

The method Valley chose was to visit a number of comparable hospitals with excellent reputations and demonstrated achievements in the areas of its interest. Our primary premise was that, since these hospitals had achieved their results independently of each other, we would find that they excelled in different ways and that much could be learned from identifying the reasons for their achievements. Our secondary premise was that, since we would be dealing with implemented rather than theoretical or untried ideas, the problem of convincing ourselves of their practicability would be reduced.

The hospitals that participated in this study are as follows:**

- Abington Memorial Hospital   Abington, Pennsylvania
- Alta Bates Hospital   Berkeley, California
- Blodgett Memorial Medical Center   Grand Rapids, Michigan
- Bryn Mawr Hospital   Bryn Mawr, Pennsylvania
- Hackensack Hospital   Hackensack, New Jersey
- Holy Spirit Hospital   Camp Hill, Pennsylvania
- Huntington Hospital   Huntington, New York
- McKay-Dee Hospital Center   Ogden, Utah
- Memorial Hospital of Du Page County   Elmhurst, Illinois
- St. Luke's Hospital   New Bedford, Massachusetts

** Throughout this book, statements about "hospitals" or "all hospitals" refer to this group.

- St. Joseph's Hospital   Tucson, Arizona
- St. Rita's Medical Center   Lima, Ohio
- Suburban Hospital   Bethesda, Maryland
- Swedish Medical Center   Englewood, Colorado
- The Valley Hospital   Ridgewood, New Jersey

In addition, we briefly visited the Northern California headquarters and Corporate headquarters of the Kaiser-Permanente Medical Care Program, both in Oakland, California.

Our visits were relatively brief — about five working days per hospital. This was ample for our purposes, given the narrowness of our focus, our search for ideas rather than details, the quality and openness of those with whom we met, the repetition of subject areas from hospital to hospital, our own familiarity with the subject matter, and the material received from each hospital in advance of our visit. In total, we interviewed more than 280 senior people individually or, in a few instances, in pairs:

- 70 well-established and respected senior admitting physicians, representing all of the major specialties
- 7 chiefs of medical staffs or directors of medical education
- 14 chief executive officers
- 22 hospital trustees
- 14 radiologists
- 13 pathologists
- 12 Utilization Review Committee chairmen (all physicians)
- 14 directors of nursing
- 14 chief financial officers or controllers
- 25 assistant hospital administrators or directors of planning
- 75 department heads (e.g., laboratory manager, operating room manager, utilization review coordinator)

The ideas and conclusions set forth in this book are drawn from the vast experience and talent of these individuals. Quotations from interviews are not cited by source in order to protect the identity of the people and their institutions.

COMMENTS ON METHOD

The approach that we took worked out well in practice:

1. The fundamental premise proved to be valid — individual hospitals have increased their capacity to admit and treat more patients,

using a variety of methods to achieve low lengths of stay and high rates of occupancy. Each hospital visited contributed ideas and techniques that were valuable. In turn, there is evidence that each hospital has opportunities to improve its own operations by incorporating techniques or programs employed elsewhere. Although there may be some absolute lower limit on length of stay, no hospital visited has yet reached it for all patient classifications, services, or diagnoses.

2. Direct, on-site observation of successful programs, procedures, etc., has great impact on the observers. The opportunity to learn firsthand of initial and lasting strengths and problems and to obtain the frank reactions of the affected parties is invaluable.

3. Many operational improvements can be achieved by methods and approaches that are already known to some members of the medical and hospital community. The biggest differences among hospitals result, not from new ideas, but from how intensively, extensively, and imaginatively known ideas and techniques are carried out. This could often be seen by comparing similar situations in different hospitals.

4. The reasons that individual hospitals have reached their present level of effectiveness and, at times, have not progressed beyond it are varied and complex. The past existence of a bed shortage for a substantial period of time is a relatively simple cause which has a variety of essentially direct, predictable effects. At the other end of the scale, the impacts of reimbursement systems, malpractice suits, the cultural characteristics of patients, and the history and traditions of the local medical staff are often subtle, strong, and contradictory. The variety and complexity of these and other factors are also clarified by contrast.

Summary of Conclusions

We began this project with the hope of identifying techniques that might stretch the bed capacity of The Valley Hospital by ten percent. We believe that we will exceed that goal. However, we also discovered (1) that both the questions and answers involved are bigger, more complex, and more subtle than we had anticipated and (2) that the contributions to be made by the medical staff must, in many instances, be as great or greater than those which can be made by the administration or board of trustees.

In substantive terms, our major conclusions are as follows:

1. Attempts to operate each individual department in a hospital at its own maximum efficiency — with relatively little regard for the effects of those policies on other departments, doctor efficiency, and patient progress — consistently have counterproductive results. These attempts become increasingly damaging as occupancy rates approach maximum capacity and lengths of stay drop. Management and medical staff policies should more directly focus on the hospital-wide impact of programs and operating procedure on capacity, efficiency, and cost. Regulatory agencies involved in rate setting, planning, and project review must be equally vigilant with respect to the hospital-wide and system-wide implications of their policies.

2. As a hospital approaches maximum occupancy and lengths of stay drop, the need for hospital/medical staff cooperation, coordination, and participative decision making increases. Hospital administrators and hospital departments make a significant difference in determining how efficiently a hospital operates as "an instrument" and how effectively it responds in a timely manner to the needs of individual members of the medical staff. The practicing physicians, in total and individually, exert an even greater influence through their direct control of the number of patients admitted to the hospital and the period of time for which they stay. However, the successful interaction between the hospital and its physicians has potentially the greatest impact on hospital operations. In short, the total is greater than the sum of the parts.

   In order to successfully manage the complex problems that result from a high-occupancy, short-stay situation, the relationship between administration and the key physicians on the medical staff must develop far more fully than the traditional, laissez-faire relationship that exists in most hospitals. This involves greater predecision identification of both internal and external aspects of a problem, greater physician input as to possible solutions and their impact, and substantial assistance from key physicians in implementing solutions and obtaining the understanding and support of their colleagues.

3. Substantial variations in lengths of stay exist for comparable diagnoses for essentially similar patients. These differences exist (1) among doctors of the same institution, (2) among institutions, and (3) among major regions of the country. Further, the performance of a given hospital with respect to one diagnosis is not necessarily indicative of its performance with respect to another, even among our selected group of outstanding hospitals.

Even a modest goal such as bringing the performance of hospitals, doctors, and diagnoses with above-average length of stay down to the median performance would produce dramatic increases in productive capacity. And, if one considers the achievement of hospitals in the broad and varied western region of the United States and uses that as a standard toward which hospitals in other regions of the country could move, the results would be even more significant.

4. There is an impressive and continuing growth in the number and complexity of the operations being carried out as one-day surgical procedures, with one hospital carrying out 45 percent of its operations on that basis. (See page 27 [Chapter II] for a respresentative listing.) Virtually all hospitals use special areas for preoperative care and recovery. Several hospitals are using dedicated operating rooms (ORs) to provide these services at a lower cost, while simultaneously freeing the regular operating room suite for major operations, simplifying scheduling, reducing the cancellation of elective cases, and achieving other benefits.

5. As lengths of stay decrease, the ability to make full use of bed capacity becomes increasingly dependent upon the availability of operating room time. A few hospitals make impressive use of extended hours on weekdays and Saturdays for elective surgery or, as discussed above, have developed surgical centers for ambulatory patients. Where these solutions prove to be impractical or undesirable, hospitals may find it necessary to eliminate an operating room bottleneck through construction.

6. All the hospitals, except one, attempt to meet peak demands by employing temporary beds amounting to between 5 and 12 percent of the medical/surgical capacity. In many instances, these are nothing more than temporary beds, used to provide care until inpatient beds are available. In several hospitals, however, necessity has been turned into a virtue as the temporary quarters have been adapted to meet the special needs of the (normally emergency) patients who occupy them.

7. Only limited efforts are being made to tap the substantial amount of off-peak time that is available on weekends and in and around holidays and vacation periods. Some hospitals, however, are doing interesting and productive things. The use of off-peak demand is a very complex issue — medically, culturally, economically, managerially, and fiscally — and deserves serious study under any program of mandated bed restrictions.

8. The various performance review programs (utilization review,

medical audit, and Professional Standards Review Organizations [PSRO] review) have had a very mixed reception, both individually and collectively. PSRO efforts are uniformly described as having results that are somewhere between counterproductive and marginally productive, whether carried out on a delegated basis or nondelegated basis. The range of reactions to utilization review and medical audit is greater — varying from essential neutrality to substantial enthusiasm and impressive achievements. The latter reaction occurred in hospitals where the efforts have strong and dedicated leadership and a focus that is both broad (in that it extends over a wide range of cases and activities) and selective (in that it focuses on problem cases, diagnoses, doctors, and situations) and constructive (in that its primary emphasis is on the identification and correction of causes rather than the prevention of abuses).

One sees numerous indications of the ability of specific doctors to make the hospital work efficiently for them, an ability that is not always present in other members of the staff. One gets the impression that, in spite of the absence of efforts to teach such efficiency, some of the better utilization review efforts may be having educative, as well as medical, results.

9. The availability of hospital-based diagnostic, treatment, and therapeutic services — as measured in terms of days and hours, complexity of tests offered, and types of patients covered — both reflects and controls a hospital's rate of occupancy and the length of stay of many of its patients. All hospitals provide the services they deem necessary to handle emergency cases on a routine or standby basis throughout the day and week. The differences, therefore, affect the coverage provided primarily for elective cases and certain patients of other categories during the days of recovery. Undoubtedly, the most critical departments are (1) the radiology department and, to a considerably lesser degree, (2) the laboratory, (3) the operating room, and (4) physical therapy. These services are substantially limited, except for emergency cases, in virtually all instances on weekday evenings and weekends. There are, however, a limited number of important, major exceptions and a sufficient number of indications that normal hours are being stretched by staggering, after-hours consultations, etc., to suggest that extensions in coverage are practical.

10. The speed of response to doctors' requests for diagnostic and other services has an important effect on length of stay. Most hospitals find preadmission testing (PAT) beneficial and use it for a high proportion of their elective cases. The time required for inpatient di-

agnostic tests often reflects the doctor's own diagnostic skills and personal organization and behavior. To the extent that response time is within the hospital's control, it normally depends on the speed with which steps other than that of making the test itself are carried out — e.g., patient transportation, transcription, the placement of test results on the patient's chart, and particularly, the reduction of delays when nothing is occurring.* A number of effective techniques, in addition to good interdepartmental coordination and departmental management, can be of help.

11. In the past ten or twenty years, there has been a great deal of discussion about the hospital's role as a part or, more properly, the hub of a health care system. For a variety of reasons, this role has been only partially realized. With one or two important exceptions, only minimal efforts have been made in prehospital areas such as preventive medicine and health education. There has been more interest in posthospital care — in part, because of the hospital's frequent inability to discharge patients no longer needing acute care. The result has been, where reimbursement policies make it feasible, the acquisition and operation of nursing homes, the development of effective hospital-based home care departments or of effective relationships with external agencies, and the creation of hospice programs. There is substantial evidence that, given reasonable reimbursement, these programs would be expanded with considerable advantage in terms of bed availability.

12. There is a definite relationship between the managerial policies and actions of a hospital and the reimbursement system under which it operates. It is unrealistic to expect otherwise. Yet it also is impressive to see the number of instances in which hospitals with available bed capacity are still reducing their already low lengths of stay and encouraging further efforts in that direction.

It is hard to recognize a lack of efforts to eliminate permitted costs or practices resulting from the absence of positive incentives to do so. And in virtually all of the reimbursement systems (with the probable exception of health maintenance organization [HMO] systems) they clearly do not exist. What can be seen are the negative effects of underreimbursement and rate review. Prime examples of this are:

---

* See Chapter III, section on "Radiology Services," for a full discussion of the implications of delays in handling patients.

    a. Inadequate Medicaid nursing home payments that force the hospital to retain patients at a very high cost to the health care system.

    b. Inadequate payments for services rendered on an outpatient basis that are fully covered for inpatients.

    c. Rate review that concentrates heavily on individual cost centers to the detriment of overall hospital effects.

13. HMOs and other organizations in which doctors or other group purchasers have a significant economic incentive have an important impact on patients, doctors, and hospitals.

14. It is evident, on the basis of the experience of hospitals with high rates of occupancy and limited opportunities to accommodate more doctors and patients through reductions in length of stay, that some way must be found to limit admissions to the medical staff. Otherwise, with the ability to expand closed off by regulatory action, some combination of chaos and tension will result to the inevitable disadvantage of patient, doctor, and hospital. The few tentative attempts we encountered and the few court cases that are available do not recognize the freeze on hospital capacity that has been externally imposed. It should not be the responsibility of an individual hospital to proceed unguided through this situation. Rather, the American Hospital Association (AHA), the American Medical Association (AMA), the Department of Health and Human Services (HHS), or some other authorized body should deal with the problem.

15. There are many reasons for seeking to have both a low length of stay and a high rate of occupancy. Some of these are well known; others are not. The opportunities for avoiding large capital expenditures and for lowering treatment cost per diagnosis, for example, are readily acknowledged.

Not frequently mentioned, but of substantial importance in today's environment, is the reduction of financial risk. A hospital with unfavorable occupancy/length of stay performance faces the possibility of a substantial loss of income and an increase in unoccupied beds. These effects can result rather quickly from changes in reimbursement systems, the tighter direct regulation of patient stays, or the introduction into the area of HMOs or similar organizations on an extensive scale. Even a low length of stay/high occupancy hospital will not be immune to the effects of a large increase in available beds in other hospitals in its area, but its problems will be minimal by comparison.

ORGANIZATION OF THE BOOK

During the course of our survey, we developed the following definition of what an efficient hospital should be. It is one that has:

a. the capacity to respond quickly, properly, and economically with appropriate services and to provide the setting and support physicians require for prompt patient care;
b. physicians on its medical staff who aggressively use the facilities and services of the hospital and those found elsewhere in the community, and who use them properly and economically; and
c. the ability to adapt to changes and influence forces in its environment effectively and expeditiously.

The remainder of this book, presented in six major sections, reflects the many and varied ways in which individual hospitals are attempting to conform to this definition. The six sections are divided into chapters as follows:

II.–III. Making the Hospital an Efficient Instrument
    IV. Facilitating the Efficient Use of the Hospital by Attending Physicians
     V. Making Appropriate Use of Alternatives to Hospital Care: the Effective Use of Other Community Resources
    VI. Informing, Influencing, and Adapting to the Hospital's Environment
   VII. Census Control through Medical Staff Regulation and Limitation

These sections contain a discussion of ideas, policies, and techniques that meet two criteria. First, they are found by individual hospitals to be particularly effective. Second, they stand out either because they are different or are applied so as to produce considerably above-average results. The book does not contain a summary of practices except where that information provides the necessary background for our comments.

A concluding chapter contains a series of questions which we believe can be of significant value to any individual hospital wishing to assess its own programs and policies. Two appendixes, containing items of interest, complete the book.

II

Making the Hospital an Efficient Instrument through Policies and Practices Concerning Capacity, Scheduling, Cancellations, and Discharges

A hospital's ability to provide maximum services is dependent, in part, on its skill in solving the kinds of problems with which hotels, airlines, and others with essentially fixed capacities and fluctuating demands are familiar — meeting the peaks and leveling out the valleys. The major differences that hospitals face lie in (1) the unpredictability of some of that demand and the priority accorded to emergency patients, and (2) the relatively limited options that hospitals have available.

Within these limitations, a number of effective and, at times, ingenious policies and practices are possible. Some that we encountered are discussed in this section under the following headings:

- Maximizing the Availability of Beds during Periods of Peak Demand
- Off-peak Utilization
- Outpatient or One-day Surgery
- Scheduling, Admitting, and Cancelling
- Discharge Management

It will be noted that in this and other sections of the book, we have assumed that the construction of additional beds is not a practical alternative for regulatory reasons. However, since many of the comments apply with equal force in the absence of such limitations, given the high cost of constructing and operating underutilized beds, the discussion has rather general applicability.

Maximizing the Availability of Beds
During Periods of Peak Demand

Coping with Peak Demands

"Hello, Mrs. Smith? This is the hospital. I'm sorry, but we've had to cancel your admission and surgery tomorrow because of a lack of beds. Please call your doctor to reschedule." This message is repeated thousands of times across the country during times of peak occupancy. Nobody likes it. Patients must alter personal and business plans and gear themselves up emotionally a second time for the trauma of surgery; surgeons have their schedules disrupted; the hospital suffers a loss of productivity in the operating room; and a deterioration of community relationships results.

One way of improving the supply of available inpatient beds — short of construction — is to reduce the demand for those beds — to eliminate unnecessary admissions, to hasten discharge, and to expand the use of outpatient services. But even assuming this has been accomplished and that as much of the demand as is practical has been diverted into periods of lower demand, peaks can be expected that will at times exceed the nominal capacity of the hospital. A number of methods can be and are employed to increase the availability of beds during these periods. These range from simple "capacity stretching" through the temporary use of extra beds in treatment or multi-bed rooms, to specialized holding areas, to mixed nursing units, to specialized areas that smooth admissions and discharge procedures, etc.

Temporary Beds

Little needs to be said about the use of temporary beds in corridors, solaria, semiprivate rooms, treatment rooms, etc. Our survey confirms that this procedure is widespread, even in institutions that have developed other more sophisticated mechanisms for managing their census. Temporary beds employed at times of peak demand range from 5 to 12 percent of the normal or licensed capacity of medical/surgical beds.

Only a few of the participating hospitals place patients in the halls. Many refuse to do so as a matter of policy, and those that do, use corridor beds only as a last resort. Nearly all hospitals, however, put overflow patients in treatment rooms, add a bed to semiprivate rooms, or place "boarders" in their intensive care unit (ICU) or coronary care unit (CCU) before they cancel admissions. Most patients occupying temporary beds are transferred to regular inpatient beds on the following day. Some quarters are sufficiently satisfactory and attractive, however, so that patients whose hospital stay will be short need not be moved.

Few hospitals or their patients prefer temporary beds and most regard them as somewhere between a necessary evil and a pragmatic compromise. They do, however, recognize that they are also a very cost-efficient way of coping with periods of peak demand and represent a method of increasing the total service capacity of the institution. The alternatives are the postponement and, perhaps, the loss of patient admissions or a commitment to major capital expenditures and ongoing operating expenses for additional regular beds that will be needed only a small percentage of the time.

HOLDING AREAS

As an additional method of accommodating peak patient loads, the hospitals surveyed have successfully developed several types of "holding areas," adapted to the specific purposes they are to serve. These are:

1. Emergency room (ER) holding or observation areas
2. Recovery room holding areas
3. Preoperative holding areas
4. Discharge holding areas

Each of these is designed to provide to a specific category of patients medical care that is commensurate with a patient's needs until an appropriate inpatient bed becomes necessary or available.

Emergency holding and observation areas. Four hospitals have holding and observation areas with capacities from two to ten patients. All are immediately adjacent to the ER and are specifically designed for the short-term (less than 24 hours) management of severely ill or traumatized patients on those occasions when intensive-care or coronary-care or other inpatient beds are filled to capacity. Such units are typically equipped with telemetry (monitored by the ER, CCU, or ICU staffs) and staffed by Emergency Room nurses.

Patients needing inpatient beds are given top priority for transfer to an appropriate inpatient bed (usually within 12–24 hours). However, in at least one facility, there have been occasions where individual patients have remained in the ER holding area for more than 48 hours. By contrast, some patients — especially those arriving as the result of accidents — are found, after observation, not to require further treatment and are sent home.

The institutions operating these areas are committed to their continuing use. They state that, first, they provide the institution with the ability to add to its capacity without the construction or permanent staffing of regular beds. More important, the physicians contend that while the use of such an area causes certain staffing problems for nursing and certain patient management problems for the attending physician, the care received by these patients is nearly as good as that received in the special care units during the day and is clearly preferable to placing critically ill patients elsewhere in the hospital, particularly at night, when most of the patients arrive.

In one institution — a designated trauma center in an Emergency Medical Services (EMS) system — the ER holding area also serves as the place where seriously ill patients can be appropriately cared for and monitored while they await transfer to another hospital or specialized facility.

Recovery room holding areas. The concept of holding a limited number of patients in the recovery room following surgery, while not broadly used, has been successfully employed as a part of an overall bed-use strategy. Patients are admitted routinely for surgery. However, if the demand for beds is unusually high on the day of their surgery, admitting will reassign their bed to an incoming patient, and the particular patient who has gone to the operating room will be held in the recovery room until another bed becomes available. The hospital must absorb the costs of a patient transfer and of overnight staffing of the recovery room. However, accepting another admission more than offsets the additional costs and provides service that otherwise would not be available.

Patients selected for this procedure tend to be those who have had serious surgery and who would be most apt to benefit from the ready availability of monitoring and recovery equipment and the close attention provided by a low staff-to-patient ratio. In no case are patients held longer than overnight in the recovery room. They frequently are patients who otherwise might have spent the night in the intensive care unit. The following day, these patients are given priority over all incoming admissions for bed assignments.

Postpartum obstetrical patients are also held overnight in the obstetrics recovery room of some hospitals when other beds on the maternity unit are full. So long as the husband is given access to this room, few patient complaints result from this practice. Women who are retained in the obstetrics recovery room are given priority over incoming admissions for bed assignments.

Preoperative holding areas. The most frequently observed type of holding area is the preoperative area. In some cases, these areas are also used during the day as staging and recovery areas for surgical outpatients. However, in other hospitals, the preoperative holding areas are specifically designed for patients who are to undergo major surgery the following day and who require limited preparation or minimal nursing care the previous night. Some institutions also admit so-called "A.M. admissions" to this type of area to avoid the disruption of regular nursing units that this type of admission often causes. (See page 30 for a complete discussion of A.M. admissions.)

Because these preoperative patients have limited needs, the staffing can be kept to a minimum and the physical area designed so as to maximize the number of patients. Depending upon the regulations of individual states, these beds may or may not be classified as licensed inpatient beds.

Discharge holding areas. Patients who cannot or do not leave the hospital when they are medically able to do so deprive those seeking admission of a bed by continuing to occupy their room. A special group of these patients are those who do not leave the hospital on the day of discharge as early as regulations require and, in the absence of an alternative, stay in their rooms until someone appears to take them home. In one hospital with a strong utilization review program, a recent (1978) study identified 121 such patients in an eight-week period.

The obvious answer might seem to be to enforce discharge regulations more rigidly. However, this is difficult, and all hospitals report they have been no more than partially successful in doing so. It is worth noting that one hospital moved its discharge time from 11 A.M. to 10 A.M. and achieved some improvement in average departure time.

We noted that another interesting way of coping with the problem of the lingering patient is the creation of a special discharge holding area. Two hospitals have recently begun to provide this service, while a third plans to do so in the near future. It functions as follows:

> Once a patient has been clinically discharged, the floor nurses immediately inquire if the patient might have difficulty in making the necessary arrangements for discharge prior to a fixed hour (usually 11 A.M.). If problems exist and the physician does not specify otherwise, the patient is told that he or she

will be relocated "at no extra charge" (patients uniformly do not pay for their last day anyway!) to a specific area to await whoever is picking them up. In one hospital, patients (usually three or less) are placed in a holding area near the admitting lobby where they are observed by the nurses performing the Preadmission testing function. In another example, an RN is assigned to the discharge holding area as part of her responsibility. Patients are provided with television, cards, magazines, access to bathrooms, and appropriate meals.

MIXED NURSING UNITS

Each of the hospitals has, at one time or another, come to grips with the issue of specialized nursing units. All hospitals specialize to the extent of having specific units for the ICU and/or CCU, pediatrics, obstetrics (with or without "clean" gynecology), and psychiatry. It is in the further specialization of nursing units — for orthopedics, urology, ophthalmology, general surgery, etc. — that controversy exists. It is generally agreed that specialized nursing units provide patients with a nursing staff that is well practiced in caring for the particular problems of that unit's primary patients and knows the treatment practices and idiosyncrasies (including writing) of individual physicians. Physicians also normally prefer it for the foregoing reasons and because, with all of their patients on one floor, they save time and effort in making their rounds.

Reactions of nurses are said to be more varied. Some prefer specialization while many others enjoy the broader experience of handling a variety of patients or avoiding the continuing physical or emotional problems associated with specific diagnoses. Mixed units also permit greater interchangeability and flexibility in nursing staff assignments and may contribute to a reduction in nursing care hours per patient day.

From the standpoint of bed availability, most of the arguments are on the side of general purpose units. Both theory and practical experience support the conclusion that nonspecialized nursing units permit higher occupancy levels and reduce the risks of patient nonaccommodation. The admitting office simply has greater flexibility in the assignment of patients. In spite of the fact that, under peak conditions, virtually all beds become at least temporarily interchangeable, under near-peak conditions the problems of saving beds for special purposes become very difficult to handle. Institutions that have switched to mixed units feel that the net effect has been positive. They state, however, that the process of change has not been an easy one. Physicians, in particular, have preferred specialized nursing units and have agreed to change only when the administration and medical staff leadership have been able to demonstrate to attending physicians that the advantages of increased bed availability substantially outweigh those resulting from the retention of specialized units.

Instances were observed where mixing has been successfully carried to the point where medical/surgical patients are freely admitted to psychiatric, pediatric, and gynecological units at times of high occupancy. Licensure regulations will determine whether this is permitted in specific states, but, based on the experience of these hospitals, no significant medical problems exist.

EXPANDING ICU/CCU BED CAPACITY

Several hospitals have expanded their ability to handle ICU/CCU patients by the development of units that enable patients to move through an intermediate stage of care before being transferred to regular inpatient beds. These stepped-down units are usually, but not always, physically adjacent to the ICU units and CCU units. The more important requirements are (1) that they be adequately equipped with monitoring equipment that can be satisfactorily be read by nurses in the stepped-down unit, or by telemetry in the ICU/CCU units, or by both, and that (2) fast and competent response is available in the case of emergencies.

While the length of stay in this unit naturally varies considerably, it approximates the time spent in the ICU/CCU.

EMERGENCY SAFETY LEVELS

All hospitals have established their own policies as to the number of beds that will be held available for overnight emergency admissions, or they are restricted to the number set by relevant state regulations. Such beds are held in reserve after 3:00 P.M. each day in order to assure that emergency patients admitted before the following morning can be accommodated. Several hospitals not only save a given number of medical/surgical beds (usually 2 to 4 percent of total capacity) but also beds in specialized areas (particularly mixed obstetrics/gynecology [OB/GYN] units where as much as 10 to 15 percent of the available capacity is held in reserve daily). Strict and constant utilization of these types of safety factors will inevitably reduce the hospital's ability to achieve maximum occupancy, even in times of peak demand, and will lead to excessive cancellations of elective patients.*

---

* As reported by David H. Stimson and Ruth H. Stimson in *Operations Research in Hospitals: Diagnosis and Prognosis* (Chicago: Hospital Research and Educational

It appears to us that most safety factors, particularly those established by state regulation:

a. are too high on a statistical basis,
b. fail to consider the availability of alternative regular and temporary beds, stretchers, etc.,
c. are too rigidly employed, and
d. do not consider the use of other hospitals as "layoff" facilities.

Some hospitals have reduced the self-established or mandatory safety levels by demonstrating that they are excessive on the basis of experience and need, taking their own surrounding hospitals into account. Others have reduced the need for saving licensed beds by temporarily placing emergency patients in a variety of temporary beds and holding areas, "playing the float" of late discharges to a greater degree,** and/or considering that inpatient safety beds are essentially interchangeable except for medical reasons. Two institutions claim that careful management of the daily number of scheduled elective admissions (following the procedures described on pages 28–30), combined with a willingness to place an occasional patient in a treatment room or hold a patient in the ER, pending the availability of a regular bed, helps to avoid elective admissions cancellations completely while minimizing or eliminating their safety beds for emergencies.

LAYOFF ARRANGEMENTS

We expected and, in fact, did find that neighboring hospitals have developed informal cooperative arrangements, in which ambulance corps and police departments are also involved, to divert incoming patients to hospitals with available beds when others are at or near their capacity. We hoped also to find layoff arrangements which went beyond this usual

---

Trust, 1972), p. 16, a study of emergency admissions by Newell, using the Poisson distribution, indicated that when the average demand for emergency admissions was between one and thirty per day, only two beds more than average were needed to satisfy the demand 95 percent of the time.

** In such instances, hospitals hold few, if any, beds at 3:00 P.M. and simply count on the fact that late discharges and deaths will usually provide a sufficient number of beds for after-hours emergency admissions. Where there are a large number of late discharges, it is highly probable this technique will succeed.

relationship, overcoming the barrier to maximizing area-wide bed availability that exists when a doctor loses his regular patient unless he is a member of the medical staff of the receiving hospital. In this respect, we were partially successful, for four institutions have developed limited mechanisms that encourage physicians to use an alternative facility when their normally preferred hospital is fully occupied. These mechanisms are as follows:

1. One hospital formally consolidated its medical staff with a neighboring institution in 1972, following several years of broadly based discussions and the development of detailed bylaws for a combined staff. The final decision was made with the unanimous approval of all physicians at both hospitals.*** These institutions retain separate corporate identities, separate boards of trustees and separate administrations and, in fact, compete with each other on many levels.

    With a single staff, a single physician director of medical affairs coordinating their Interhospital Education Association, and joint educational and departmental meetings, these institutions have eliminated the organization barriers that normally keep physicians from moving freely between two hospitals. Nonetheless, while these two hospitals have also successfully consolidated several inpatient services (pediatrics and neurosciences at one hospital and obstetrics and cardiology at the other), the respective admitting offices expect the physician or his office to take the initiative and try the other hospital when beds are short.

2. At another institution, located in a municipality with one other hospital, the physicians have almost unanimously decided to join both staffs. While each physician has a hospital of preference, the generally high levels of occupancy experienced by both hospitals make it necessary for physicians to admit an occasional patient to the other hospital. The institutions have responded by approving a number of joint medical staff committees and departmental meetings in order to minimize the duplication of administrative and educational activities to which each physician is subjected. There is not, however, a formal mechanism for laying off patients during those few times when only one hospital is full to capacity. This is, perhaps,

---

*** The Estes Park Institute has published a book by Zeke Scher describing this consolidation, entitled *The Denver Connection* (Estes Park Institute, Englewood, Colo., 1976).

quite understandable, since hospitals in a small geographic area tend to reach peak levels of occupancy simultaneously, thereby minimizing the advantages that layoff arrangements might otherwise provide. In addition, however, it is evident that competition for patients and doctors is a factor.

3. Physicians at a third institution, located in a municipality with three hospitals, have, of necessity, developed their own informal layoff situation. Almost all physicians in this municipality are affiliated with one of the two larger hospitals as well as with the smallest of the three. Because it is older, smaller, and somewhat less sophisticated in its scope of services, this third hospital is least likely to be the first choice of the admitting physicians except for medical cases. It is, however, an entirely acceptable alternative for most other services. Because overall occupancy at both of the larger hospitals (including the one we visited) is high and because there is little crossover of medical staffs between these two hospitals, there is a fairly high and consistent demand for beds at the third hospital.

   Hospital administrators were quick to acknowledge the existence and benefits of this informal layoff mechanism and indicated that all three hospitals are in close touch about bed availability when occupancy is high. Nonetheless, while the hospitals may agree to a redirection of ambulance cases, they have not attempted to develop any mechanism that would redirect previously scheduled elective admissions.

4. A slightly different variation of a similar theme exists at a fourth institution located in a suburban county with a large number of physicians and several competing institutions. Here the hospital and the county medical society have taken steps to assure that physicians who normally practice at a given hospital can gain temporary privileges elsewhere, good for single admissions, when beds are tight at their own primary hospital. The institution we visited has a quick and easy method of granting temporary privileges for single admissions to physicians accredited by neighboring institutions.

   Because the bed supply in the area is neither inadequate nor excessive, the use of multiple institutions by physicians has helped to reduce the risks of patient nonaccommodation. The hospital itself, however, has not developed a formal mechanism for encouraging patient layoffs, and, in fact, foresees greater interhospital competition in the future.

In sum, what we had assumed to be a problem of patient loss by a physician, turned out only in part to be that. We also found, first, that a severe handicap to the area-wide utilization of beds often exists because of the difficulties involved in obtaining and maintaining membership on more than one hospital staff (particularly because of the educational and service obligations that are assumed). Second, we encountered an apparent and understandable reluctance — based on economic and competitive factors — among hospitals to develop interhospital referral/layoff arrangements for other than emergency cases. And, third, we found that a number of doctors strongly preferred to practice at one hospital because of their feelings about the interdependence of physicians — the subtle existence of an informal but effective group practice that exists within a close-knit group of physicians who continuously practice together as one medical staff.

OFF-PEAK UTILIZATION

All of the hospitals have substantial unused capacity during weekends and certain school vacations and around certain national and religious holidays. During these periods, occupancy falls from a normal level of about 90 percent to 70–80 percent or less, or in similar proportion in hospitals with other normal levels of occupancy. The problem is accentuated by short lengths of stay, as the probability of fully handling a patient increases in the Monday–Friday period.

Hospitals with normally *low* rates of occupancy often adapt to the situation by reducing weekend activities as much as possible, deliberately concentrating on the Monday–Friday period to reduce costs and provide an "affordably high" level of care. Under such an approach, the hospital maintains an ability to respond to emergencies, but provides other in-patients with little more than custodial care, with little or no medical progress, during weekends. Hospitals with *intermediate* and *high* rates of occupancy are less able to use such a strategy, because of the negative effect it has on length of stay and occupancy. Hospitals with high demand must make better use of weekends to accommodate doctors and patients. Those with intermediate demand have more options available, but they, too, can rarely afford to provide only custodial care on weekends. How much care is the question. The facts are, of course:

1. that emergencies are not confined to the Monday–Friday period,
2. that the condition of patients already in the hospital makes the weekend discharge of all patients unthinkable,
3. that the hospital finds itself with an obligation to provide a substantial capacity for weekend service that is, in considerable part, underused and, in considerable part, not fully satisfied, and

4. that, when a capacity to serve emergency and continuing patients is available, a capacity to handle additional elective patients also exists.

Most of the hospitals are going modestly beyond providing a custodial level of care on weekends, but only a few are making what could fairly be described as a substantially greater use of that period. None have seriously attempted to cope with the drop in census related to school vacations and holidays except by adjusting their staffing complement.

Most of the increase in weekend use that exists has been brought about by one or more of the following approaches:

1. Opening one or more operating rooms for elective cases on Saturday morning or all day Saturday. (In the maximum instance, one hospital provides 75 percent of its normal operating capacity for the entire day.)
2. Providing a substantial range of radiological and laboratory services to elective patients on Saturday morning and, in several institutions, throughout the entire weekend.
3. Handling admissions and operations during the week so that a greater number of patients would be in recovery stages on weekends.

Historically, increases in weekend activity have originated primarily from shortages in beds, operating room time, etc., that more or less forced extended hours of use. Of minor but slightly growing importance has been patient convenience and interhospital competition. Of substantial interest is the fact that once hours are extended, they are rarely reshortened.

The reasons that low weekend demand persists are relatively consistent:

1. Most practicing physicians and hospital-based doctors want their free days to fall on the weekend for "quality of life" reasons. (Apparently, hospital-based employees can be hired in adequate quantity and quality on weekends, although, in some areas, only at premium salaries.)
2. Many, if not most, doctors feel that hospital-based services are incomplete or less-than-first class on weekends and thus are not suited for the needs of their patients at certain stages of their diagnosis and treatment.
3. Hospitals and hospital-based physicians — in a classic "chicken/egg" situation — are reluctant or unwilling to expand the hours or increase the costs of providing service in the absence of a strong indication that the demand exists.

4. As a matter of medical staff policy, newly admitted physicians and other categories of doctors are not forced to accept weekend admissions or operating room times nor given special priorities if they do so.

5. In all but a relatively small minority of cases, it is not currently possible to provide either the doctor or the patient with an economic incentive to use off-peak periods.

Under these circumstances, it would seem that — barring an extreme bed shortage, regulatory edict, or the like — increases in weekend use (and the extension of hours on weekdays) will be gradual and incremental. Thus, steps taken by some of the hospitals we visited should be of interest.

AVAILABILITY OF ANCILLARY DEPARTMENT SERVICES

All hospitals admit emergency patients throughout the weekend and make a major effort to provide them with the diagnostic and other ancillary services they require. The reduced availability of such services does not, therefore, affect such patients, but rather it affects (1) the admission of elective and, in some cases, urgent patients whom doctors will not admit because of an inability to make adequate progress in diagnosis and/or treatment and (2) the progress of similar patients who are already in the hospital.

In most instances, the diagnostic services provided by the laboratory and radiology departments, the services of the operating room staff and/ or the therapeutic activities of the physical therapy department are involved. In the next chapter, the text and the tables on pages 44, 45, 46, and 65 provide more information on the scheduled hours of availability of ancillary services.

Most laboratories and radiology departments provide a standard set of tests that can be handled at the technician level on an around-the-clock basis. It is in (1) the scope of the "standard set," (2) the classification of patients to whom these tests are available, and (3) the ability to provide the more difficult diagnostic services requiring doctor participation, that they vary considerably.

For a variety of reasons, both the hours of coverage and sophistication of services available during these hours have been increasing in recent years. Both the comments of a number of ancillary department doctors and the curent availability in hospitals (Tables III-1, 2, and 3, pages 44, 45, and 46) indicate that further increases are both possible and desirable. Usually, the extended coverage has been accomplished by staggering the work schedules of an existing panel of doctors or by supplementing the regular panel with a staff of permanent, although part-time, doctors.* Technical staff of the laboratory and radiology departments are also hired on a similar basis. It is of interest that, because of the existing need to provide basic coverage on weekends, the incremental increase required to provide further coverage is small, although the people involved require better training and tend to be less interchangeable.

The medical importance of initiating physical therapy soon after an accidental injury, a cardiovascular accident, or surgery and of maintaining an uninterrupted program is set forth later. Of significance in this discussion is the unwillingness of some physicians to schedule operations on a day that will require the patient to be in the hospital when physical therapy is unavailable. Only one hospital makes such services available on weekends — a situation that one would expect will have to change with the growing realization of the importance of those treatments.

AVAILABILITY OF OPERATING ROOMS

Substantial variations were likewise found in the extent to which operating rooms are available on nights and weekends. This information is presented in Table III-4, p. 65. The fundamental trend is clearly in the direction of extended hours. It is a trend that will be inevitable — unless there is a substantial increase in operating rooms — as the length of stay (LOS) decreases and the number of operations per bed/year rises. Several hospitals provide extensive hours for elective surgery on Saturday while others are actively considering it. However, in contradiction to this trend, one institution recently terminated Saturday surgery because of a perceived lack of demand.

OPERATING ROOM SCHEDULING STRATEGIES

Some hospitals have increased the use of the hospital for weekend recovery through the manner in which they schedule operations. Several institutions deliberately schedule their more complex operations later in the week with this objective in mind. Another, by assigning certain priorities in the use of the operating rooms on Monday through Thursday, encourages the use of the operating room on Friday. Finally, hospitals with separate, dedicated one-day surgical units have found that the removal of

---

* The latter method is demonstrated by one hospital where the radiology group has hired additional physicians to cover the hours of 6:00 P.M.–11:00 P.M., seven days a week, and itself covers the daytime hours through staggered schedules.

minor operations from the main operating rooms has had the unantici-
pated effect of leveling hospital occupancy by removing the effect of the
bunching of certain types of minor surgery.

PHYSICIAN COVERAGE ON WEEKENDS

In order to provide more free time on weekends, many doctors reduce
their patient load on weekends by placing their patients in what is essentially a "holding pattern" under the surveillance of a covering doctor.
Under such a pattern, the covering doctor normally acts primarily as the
agent of the attending physician, observing the progress of the patient
under the course of treatment prescribed by the attending physician, but
not altering it in any significant manner nor taking any other significant
step except in an emergency. By a process of realistic yet circular logic,
this leads to the conclusion that, since medical actions will be limited,
having the nonemergency patient in the hospital on weekends is of sharply
reduced value.

In some instances, this pattern does not seem to exist because of two or
three, apparently common, causal factors:

1. The covering doctor is given greater authority to change the treatment and, if necessary, the diagnosis of the patient. This is usually,
   but not necessarily, done after consultation with the attending physician.
2. The covering doctor is a member of the same group or partnership
   and is in the same specialty as the attending physician.
3. The covering doctor intends to work a substantial number of hours
   on the weekend — a "full shift", if such a term can be applied to doctors — and, therefore, is prepared to spend the time required by the
   more intensive coverage.

PATIENT DESIRES

The desires of patients and their families also have some influence on
the weekend utilization of hospitals. Some prefer weekend discharges in
order to simplify the problem of transporting the patient home and to ease
the transition from hospitalization. On the other hand, others prefer to
use the hospital on weekends in order to reduce the time they are away
from work. Others are quite ambivalent about it, as is probably evidenced by the fact that most weekend discharges are only marginally
affected by patient preferences.

Clearly, during periods of bed shortages, the sheer availability of beds exerts a strong influence on when patients are — and are willing to be — admitted and discharged. In other periods, doctor practice patterns and desires and the availability of services are very significant, for virtually all the doctors with whom we spoke mentioned the patient's willingness to follow the doctor's advice in virtually all key decisions.

None of the hospitals we visited had programs intended to increase weekend utilization by influencing patient attitudes directly. As far as we can determine, few, if any, successful programs have been implemented in the country — although one possible example is the well-publicized efforts of Sunrise Hospital in Las Vegas to increase weekend admissions by lotteries for free cruises.

OUTPATIENT OR ONE-DAY SURGERY

The availability of beds for inpatients has been substantially and positively affected by the development of procedures whereby patients requiring minor surgery are operated on and returned to their homes without ever occupying regular inpatient beds. Of the hospitals surveyed, all but two had developed some type of program for the specialized management of these patients. These thirteen hospitals use a dedicated patient area where patients are admitted and prepared for surgery and to which they are returned postoperatively for recovery and same-day discharge. One of these units is more than twenty years old! In addition, some hospitals perform outpatient surgery that is so minor that the use of even this area is not required.

The number and types of patients handled in this manner vary considerably. In a few hospitals, only very minor, carefully stipulated procedures can be performed as a result of internal medical staff rulings. In others, however, the scope is very broad, reaching as high as 40–50 percent of all surgical procedures,* with as many as 60–70 percent of them being carried out under general anesthesia.

---

* A partial, representative listing of the types of cases done in these ambulatory- or minor-surgery areas is as follows:

   A. *Gynecological Cases*
      1. Dilatation and curettage with conezation or cervical biopsy
      2. Laparoscopy
      3. Hymenectomy
      4. Meatomy
      5. Laparoscopy, bilateral partial salpingectomy

As the administrator of one hospital stated, "I'm amazed at how many cases these surgeons are now doing on an ambulatory basis. Specialists who said they'd never use it are some of our biggest users.... When we started out, the orthopedists couldn't think of one thing they could do there. Now, hardly a day goes by but that two or three orthopedic cases are done there."

All of the thirteen hospitals stated that their volume of one-day surgery is growing — usually rapidly — in terms of numbers of operations, types and range of operations, and complexity. They find that they attract patients from hospitals not offering the service and that it is both offensively and defensively of competitive importance insofar as patients, doctors, and hospital are concerned. It is also important in reducing both facility construction costs and operating costs.

Operationally, one-day surgery has other attractions. The stretcher beds in the dedicated patient area are rarely counted as beds for licensure purposes. They occupy far less space than inpatient beds and require less in the way of toilet and other facilities. They make effective use of the nursing staff; they permit rapid housekeeping to prepare the stretcher for

---

   B. *Cysto Cases*
      1. Standard male and female cystos
      2. Cysto with retrograde pyelogram
      3. Circumcision
   C. *Other*
      1. Extraction impacted wisdom teeth
      2. Breast reconstruction
      3. Debridement, burn with possible skin graft
      4. Excision deep lymph nodes
      5. Dermabrasion, face
      6. Scaroplasty tenolysis
      7. Excision, various lesions
      8. Rectal biopsy
      9. Tendon repairs, hand
    10. Cataract removal
    11. Excision, breast lump (suspected to be benign)
    12. Fracture reductions
    13. Tonsillectomies (selected adult)
    14. Invasive needle biopsies
    15. Hernia repair, pediatric and adult

In 1975, Alfred S. Frobese, M.D., discussed the wide scope of possibilities for ambulatory surgery ("A Surgeon's View of Ambulatory Surgery," Chapter 6, in *Ambulatory Surgical Centers*, ed., Thomas R. Donovan, Ph.D., Germantown, Md.: Aspen Systems Corp., 1976).

additional use, etc. Finally, they greatly facilitate scheduling (1) by making it essential to assign one-day surgical patients only to an area rather than a bed, (2) by reducing the number of patients who must be handled through the more complex inpatient scheduling process, and (3) by encouraging the multiple use of stretcher beds to a degree that would not be practical with inpatient facilities (one hospital frequently uses the same stretcher for two operations and one therapeutic or diagnostic procedure requiring some preparation and or recovery in the same day).

Dedicated operating rooms, such as are in use in three hospitals, also affect the use of beds and stretchers, primarily by freeing the major operating rooms for major surgery and by making sure that those coming for minor surgery will not delay elective major surgery nor have their own (minor) operations postponed or delayed. Dedicated operating rooms are discussed at greater length in the section in Chapter III titled, "Operating Rooms."

Experience in the institutions with dedicated one-day operating rooms has shown not only that the census in the rest of the hospital remains constant or increases during the week but also that census fluctuations on weekends are less dramatic. The reason is clear — with more beds and operating time available for patients requiring major surgery throughout the week, a higher proportion will be patients who will need to remain in the hospital on weekends. This positive impact on weekend occupancy is a major advantage of a well-developed, one-day-surgery program.

It is evident that the development of both a dedicated area for ambulatory patients and dedicated operating rooms requires the greatest commitment by the hospital. On the basis of our observations, it also seems to provide the greatest potential return.

SCHEDULING, ADMITTING, AND CANCELLING

Probably no areas of hospital management have attracted as much attention or been as heavily researched as the dual functions of scheduling a patient for admission and making the related room assignment. In recent years, many studies have sought to establish mathematical and statistical methods for assuring that inpatient beds and operating rooms achieve their maximum rate of use with a minimum level of patient turnaway or nonaccommodation. Many studies have resulted in complex computer-simulation models; however, as Stimson and Stimson* have noted, these models have not fared well when actually implemented.

---

* David H. Stimson and Ruth H. Stimson, *Operations Research in Hospitals: Diagnosis and Prognosis* (Chicago: Hospital Research and Educational Trust, 1972).

The hospitals we visited do not use such models. They rely on their own practical experience and that of other hospitals and on a certain amount of logic-based, trial-and-error experimentation. Approximately one-half of the hospitals visited presently have, or had previously faced, weekday requirements for beds that chronically exceed bed capacity. All hospitals, moreover, have temporary peaks during which this is a problem. In addition, because of the costs of significant fluctuations in daily census, all institutions take an active interest in methods that might help to smooth the peaks and valleys of census fluctuation. Interesting techniques observed at the hospitals visited fall into three major categories of activity:

a. scheduling of admissions,
b. cancellation of patients, and
c. room assignments.

SCHEDULING PATIENTS FOR ADMISSION

The majority of hospitals divide patient admissions into two or more categories and handle each category in a different manner. At a minimum, hospitals divide patients into "elective," or schedulable, and "emergency," or nonschedulable, categories. Most also include "urgent" as an intermediate category. In two instances, we found patients divided into a greater number of categories; however, these are primarily subtle gradations of the foregoing that have little impact on the institution's actual scheduling strategy or the methods employed to assign beds.

None of the hospitals visited has developed a sophisticated mathematical model or procedure for predicting the number and types of emergency admissions that would be requested on a given day. Instead, most have information on the average daily number of emergency admissions, which they mentally adjust and use as a guideline. All hospitals assume, until it is proven otherwise, that they can accommodate all emergency admissions and, therefore, focus most of their scheduling efforts on the manipulation of elective and urgent admissions. Basic scheduling strategies include the following:

1. At least four institutions project either their combined adult/pediatric census or combined daily admissions for the upcoming two-week period. Two of the institutions project each category individually and update the projections daily. These projections are made internally without the aid of a computer and are based on historical trends, projected changes in total patient volume, and an acknowledgment of the impact of holidays and school vacations. In every instance in which these projections have been used, the admitting

supervisor indicated that they have been helpful in minimizing patient scheduling problems.

In one eastern institution, for example, the total projected daily admissions are broken down and allocated to four classifications of patients (emergency, urgent, semi-urgent, and elective). Based upon past experience, the total number of possible admissions for a given day are apportioned among these categories. The people doing the scheduling of elective cases are, therefore, given a cutoff number after which physicians' offices are discouraged from booking further elective admissions for that particular day. The admitting supervisor in this institution feels that this system allows the hospital to distribute the patient load more evenly throughout the week, and that it has had a clearly demonstrable, positive impact on patient cancellations. In January, 1978 (two months before the system was initiated), the hospital was forced to cancel 453 previously scheduled admissions because of a lack of beds. In January, 1979, the institution had the same level of demand for beds but cancelled only 54 patients. The admitting supervisor anticipates that greater physician understanding and further refinements in the system (which still permits physicians — at a greater risk of cancellation — to schedule elective patients after the cutoff number has been reached) will allow them to approach the point where patient cancellations are a fairly rare occurrence. This is of obvious benefit to the physicians who no longer run a major risk of patient cancellation at all times. Now that risk is effectively limited to those times when a physician is willing to chance the booking of a case after the cutoff number is reached.

Other institutions with similar systems also find that the use of day-specific cutoff points for elective admissions aids their efforts to level overall occupancy and minimizes cancellation problems. As far as we could determine, in every case the cutoff points for elective admissions exclude patients destined for specialized units with traditionally lower occupancy (pediatrics, OB/GYN mixed floors, psychiatry).

2. While the previously described strategy is designed to minimize the risk of cancellation while maintaining a relatively consistent level of occupancy, other institutions use systems directed much more specifically at maximizing occupancy. At one institution, for example, the system involves a deliberate policy of overbooking, followed by a significant number of patient cancellations. Most often, however, the solution is to increase bed capacity temporarily by a modest amount above the hospital's rated capacity and to employ other

"bed-expanding" techniques. In virtually every institution, temporary beds, located in treatment rooms, solariums, corridors, etc., are used before an elective patient is cancelled. And, in others seeking to maximize occupancy, beds set aside or reserved for late emergencies are managed with special care. In fact, two high-occupancy hospitals had not cancelled a single patient in years, largely because both had the capability and the willingness to enlarge their capacity on a short-term basis by more than twenty beds located in treatment rooms, solaria, and holding areas in the emergency room.

3. In at least three institutions, A.M. admissions are used extensively. In this system, patients who are scheduled for admission for surgery arrive at the hospital early on the morning of surgery, are "admitted" to a stretcher, and, while in surgery or recovery, are assigned a bed previously occupied by a morning discharge.

   Some hospitals do not like A.M. admissions and discourage their use, citing the following:
   a. a loss of revenue under certain reimbursing mechanisms, found particularly in the East,
   b. the extra workload that is placed on nursing stations by A.M. admissions at a time when those nurses are already busy, unless additional staff is made available on the unit or in another preoperative department (e.g., one-day surgery), and
   c. the limited time available to anesthesiologists to assure themselves that the patient has not eaten, can tolerate general anesthesia, etc.

   Hospitals making use of A.M. admissions, while acknowledging these problems, believe they have been overcome to a point where they are more than outweighed by the advantages to the patient, doctor, and hospital.

4. Another system, used at one hospital that we visited and at others in its area, is designed to minimize the abuse of the emergency classification by either doctors or patients at times of peak occupancy. (In many institutions, this abuse was described as a frequent source of frustration and as a problem that resulted in an unnecessarily large number of elective patient cancellations.)

   When the institution reaches the point where eight or fewer empty medical/surgical beds (including the ICU and CCU) are available, it automatically goes on "Triage." The admitting office immediately notifies the chairman of the Utilization Review Committee who, in turn, does two things. First, he directs the utilization review department to begin identifying those patients who are the most logical candidates for discharge and to contact their attending physicians. Second, he authorizes the emergency room physicians on duty to review all patients to be admitted as emergencies. During Triage, no physician may admit an emergency patient without the approval of an emergency room physician. According to both the chief of staff and the emergency room director in that institution, this practice has been well accepted and is, in fact, now virtually a pro forma exercise. By the time the bed situation is tight, nearly all of the physicians know about it and few are likely to run the risk of attempting to fool the emergency room physician and risk the embarrassment of rejection. Commenting on the Triage system, the Chief of Staff at this hospital said: "It works very well. . . . Everybody gets very attuned to it, and. . .sort of automatically throttles back a notch or two, and we start pushing patients out a little bit faster."

5. Another scheduling problem frequently encountered by hospitals results from the ability of certain surgical specialists to book their cases well in advance. As mentioned in our discussion of the operating room, this consistently gives them first choice of prime operating room times unless they are otherwise restricted. By the same token, it gives these specialists a disproportionate ability to control bed use and occupancy levels, especially in institutions where patients are generally placed in specialized units.

In order to make the best use of their own time, these surgeons tend to schedule as many cases as possible on the same day, usually at the beginning of the week. Then, since the various eye surgeons all make similar plans, for example, the hospital faces a situation in which all of the eye patients are being admitted for surgery on Monday and Tuesday of each week. Not only do these patients disproportionately control the operating room schedule on those days, but their pattern of bed use is disruptive. All of them enter the hospital at the same time, recover postsurgically and are discharged two to four days later. By the end of the week, the nursing unit specializing in eye cases is either empty or must be used for other types of patients. However, since the cycle will normally be repeated the following week, other patients in the unit (assuming it is specialized) must be transferred or discharged in order to make room for the new eye patients. Accordingly, the hospital either faces low average occupancy in that unit or constant disruption and transfer of patients.

Two hospitals visited have resolved this problem by placing daily limitations on the number of admissions permitted by certain subspecialties. Although unpopular with the specialists, these limitations have succeeded in minimizing the problem described above.

6. Another apparently successful attempt to manipulate overall institutional occupancy by increasing weekend occupancy was observed at an eastern hospital. This facility has adjusted its surgery booking mechanism in order to encourage physicians to schedule longer-stay patients for surgery later in the week. This, in turn, means that those patients will remain in the hospital over the weekend and most probably be discharged early the following week. (This hospital appeared to be more successful than any other in the study in maintaining a high level of occupancy on the weekends. That the medical staff at this hospital is organized almost exclusively in single specialty groups may facilitate this practice since individual members have both the right and responsibility to make medical decisions affecting any of the patients of doctors in the group during the weekend they provide scheduled coverage for the group. Decisions and actions concerning a patient's care are, therefore, made rather than delayed.)

CANCELLATION TECHNIQUES

Just as the frequency with which patients are cancelled varies widely (from 20 percent of elective bookings to none), so are there variations in the methods used to select the patients to be cancelled. Without attempting to place value judgments upon them, we will describe several of the techniques encountered:

1. In the most frequently observed situation, the person in charge of admitting establishes the number of patients to be cancelled, most often selecting them on the basis of a simple queuing system (last scheduled, first cancelled).
2. In a few instances, the patients are selected on the basis of the apparent urgency of the case and the frequency with which a particular surgeon's cases have previously been cancelled. Because this method obviously involves more judgment and is open to greater objections by physicians, the admitting officer rarely makes this decision alone, but involves either an administrator or a physician. (It is of interest that, the Kaiser-Permanente group makes strenuous efforts to avoid the cancellation of elective patients, both because of its organizational philosophy and the nature of the commitment that it feels it has made to its prepaid enrollees. When a decision about patient cancellations becomes necessary, it is made jointly by the administrator and the medical director of the facility.)
In every hospital using this or the previously described system,

efforts are made to avoid cancelling the same patient more than once. However, the extent of those efforts varies — at one hospital, patients are never cancelled twice, while at another, patients being cancelled three times is not unusual.

3. One institution effectively uses the threat of cancellation to encourage Preadmission testing (PAT). At this hospital, patients who have undergone PAT are given preferred booking and are, therefore, the last to be cancelled.

4. At another hospital, when it appears that the available beds will be insufficient to accommodate all elective admissions on a particular day, the admitting officer cancels *all* scheduled admissions and notifies the affected surgeons. It then becomes the doctor's responsibility to declare their patient(s) "urgent" and again place them on the list for admission. This procedure has a certain disruptive effect on the operating room schedule, but it appears to be accepted by the doctors and to achieve its desired result.

5. Probably the most painless form of cancellation involves A.M. admissions — already described as a scheduling technique. With this technique, the patient's arrival on the afternoon before a scheduled operation is cancelled and then reinstated for the following morning so that the operation can take place as scheduled.

ROOM ASSIGNMENT TECHNIQUES

The relative merits of specialized nursing units have been discussed in Chapter II. For present purposes, it suffices to repeat that, where the admitting office has the greatest flexibility in the assignment of beds, the effective maximum occupancy is the highest and the frequency of patient cancellation is the lowest. However, regardless of the bed classification system, several observed techniques appear to have broad applicability.

1. Most hospitals have both private and semiprivate rooms, as well as newer and older rooms. Matching patient requests with the available accommodations is a source of constant problems. At one institution, this problem had been somewhat lessened and occupancy improved by always assigning semiprivate accommodations first. Only when these are filled are private rooms assigned. Because of the relatively small number of private rooms available, patients apparently view these as more of a bonus than a right.

2. Because patients are often dissatisfied with older, less spacious, or less attractive accommodations, hospitals often make a large number of transfers. In order to minimize this, one hospital requires that

physicians write a specific order stating the medical necessity for a transfer. Since the policy was instituted some years ago, the frequency of transfers has dropped significantly.

Two institutions have attempted to encourage patients to remain in less attractive rooms by pricing them well below other accommodations. However, because of the nature of most insurance coverage, they acknowledge that this has a limited impact.

3. Perhaps the most innovative and potentially valuable technique for improving bed assignments and overall occupancy is a communications technique observed between admitting and nursing personnel in a western hospital. Dubbed the "stand-up," because it was initially held in a hallway, this meeting involves the person from the admitting office who is responsible for bed assignments and an RN representative (usually the head nurse) from each nursing unit. At 11:00 A.M. each day, they gather to discuss bed assignments and patient transfers for that day. The admitting office representative brings copies of the list of that day's scheduled admissions (showing name, age, diagnosis, physician and special information such as smoking/nonsmoking) and distributes the list to everyone. The nurses in turn inform the admitting office representative of previously unreported anticipated discharges. From the list of expected admissions, the nurses then select the patients that they will take for their unit. Their decisions are based upon their available beds and the type of patients normally accommodated on the particular nursing unit. Peer pressure and a system of rewarding head nurses for high occupancy discourage thoughts of avoiding new admissions or of taking only those of minimal difficulty.

At the same time that new patients are being assigned beds, discussions may also take place between the admitting office and nursing unit representatives concerning the transfer of patients who have been inappropriately placed. In this way, all patient placement decisions are made with a maximum amount of information. The admitting office representative makes recommendations about room assignments, but the nursing unit representatives, armed with the knowledge of how a particular patient will best fit in on the nursing unit, make the final decision. The stand-up meeting rarely takes longer than ten to fifteen minutes.

This system has been in operation for a number of years. It is well accepted by both nursing and admitting office representatives and appears to be the prime contributor to the unusually cordial relationship that exists between these two departments in this hospital. This is in direct contrast with the comment made by an associate administrator at another hospital about the relationship between admitting and nursing, who said:

> I think probably the most frustrating thing, from the standpoint of nursing, is that the units find themselves having admitting call, attempting to place someone in a room without being aware of whether the patients would be compatible. . . . I think admitting finds themselves frustrated. . . in that they feel that sometimes they are not made aware of. . . beds as soon as. . . a patient is discharged.

4. In one hospital an informal system has developed whereby, during times of critical bed shortage, a physician who desires to admit an urgent patient must first discharge an in-house patient (or arrange with another physician to have him do so). When this has been accomplished, admitting will then "trade" him the bed.

DISCHARGE MANAGEMENT

FORMAL DISCHARGE PLANNING

All hospitals carry out some sort of discharge planning, with the extent and intensity of those efforts varying primarily in relation to the importance of discharge problems in the particular hospital. Secondarily, however, they reflect the commitment to length-of-stay reduction by the hospital. In some hospitals, discharge planning is a part-time function of a single person or department but, in most, is the sole responsibility of a separately identified unit with a name such as "Community Health Services Department" or "Patient and Family Services," that stresses a role of service to the patient. For the most part, the unit is managed by a person with a master's degree in social work, with there being a trend for this to be mandated by state regulation; in other hospitals, an RN with appropriate aptitudes and experience usually occupies the position.

It seems clear that early and aggressive discharge planning has an important effect on length of stay. Moreover, while the effectiveness of discharge intervention might seem to be limited when the options available are limited, the necessity for effective discharge planning remains or increases under those circumstances.

All of the hospitals start discharge planning after the patient is admitted to the hospital — in some cases, considerably after admission. This is surprising when one considers (1) the length of time required to make certain posthospital arrangements, (2) the relatively short length of hospital stay that patients frequently require for medical reasons, and (3) the fact that certain elective operations (e.g., hip replacements) can often be timed with the patient's after-stay requirements in mind. A real and as yet unused opportunity would seem to exist to start discharge planning during the preadmission period when serious problems could be anticipated. It would be initiated by the doctor and his office or the hospital discharge planner or, preferably, both. At the least, it would establish the nature of the problems, if any, and, at best, permit their solution under less pressure over a longer period of time.

At present, the hospitals we visited are rarely, if ever, working at a preadmission level but, instead, are concerned with how early in the patient's hospitalization a discharge problem can be identified. Since discharge planning units do not have enough staff to examine all charts, they normally rely on others — usually doctors, nurses or utilization review personnel — to bring problem patients to their attention. The effectiveness of this communication varies. For this reason as well as others that will be mentioned later, the discharge planning unit is often located near and made organizationally responsible to the manager of the utilization review function or more likely, both units are made responsible to the same individual. How much this improves the situation depends, in part, on the quality of the working relationships, but even more on the scope and focus of the utilization review efforts.

By and large, however, the success of discharge planning seems not to be dependent on physical systems or the flow of information so much as upon the quality of the personal efforts and the personalities of the discharge planners. The backing they receive from the doctors and the hospital administration in dealing with patients, families, and outside institutions, and the backing they receive from the medical staff and the administration in dealing with problem doctors are also important, since obviously the leverage of the discharge planner is somewhat limited. It is of interest that both of these points were frequently made about utilization review personnel. They would seem to be at least equally appropriate with respect to discharge planning.

One gets the impression that the hospitals visited consider their discharge planning to be valuable and productive — and, by and large, to be satisfactory. Somehow, in spite of that, we have the feeling that there may be considerable room for improvement.

AVAILABILITY OF POSTDISCHARGE SERVICES

Time and again during the course of our study, we found an important and direct relationship between the availability of appropriate postdischarge services (nursing homes, visiting nurses, home health aides, homemakers, rehabilitation programs, etc.) and the ability of a hospital to achieve a low length of stay. While it is not the primary determinant of length of stay, the availability of these services has a very significant impact on hospital utilization in all areas of the country.

Nursing homes. Nursing home availability appears to be the most significant factor. In most of the eastern hospitals involved in the study, an acute shortage of nursing home beds — particularly for Medicaid patients — means that, on any given day, between 5 and 8 percent of the institution's medical/surgical beds are occupied by patients awaiting transfer to nursing homes. The contrast with western hospitals, where nursing home beds are available for all classes of patients, is dramatic.

Although the options open to a hospital to minimize this problem are few, several of the hospitals studied have taken, or are considering taking, some steps worthy of note:

1. One eastern institution, acknowledging that the area-wide supply of nursing home beds is inadequate, has taken steps to assure that its patients receive as many of these nursing home beds as possible. Its approach has been to develop close working relationships with the major nursing homes — providing educational opportunities to their employees, engaging in joint purchasing arrangements, and assisting in the development of their managerial talent. It has, in essence, developed a type of symbiotic relationship which has allowed that hospital's patients to gain some measure of preferred status.
2. Two hospitals have acquired or are considering the acquisition of nursing homes in states where the reimbursement system provides the opportunity to realize a satisfactory profit. These nursing homes, which may or may not be publicly identified with the hospital, provide guaranteed placement for the hospital's patients and, more than that, an important element in those hospital's efforts to create an integrated health care system.

    The key, of course, is the reimbursement system(s). In some states, nursing homes can and do generate a substantial return on investment when they are efficiently operated. In others, the return is more modest. But, in an unfortunately large number of other states, the reimbursement on certain types of patients — particularly Medicaid patients — is so low that a hospital-related nursing home, accepting all types of patients, will be in severe financial difficulty.

    It is of interest that hospitals with nursing homes manage and operate those homes with personnel who are not drawn from or used intermittently in the hospital, since they must compete with a preponderance of homes without hospital affiliations and with reimbursing systems that are based on their levels of care and cost.

3. The need for *hospitals* to support adequate reimbursement for nursing homes that are not owned by the hospital seems to be both obvious and unrecognized. Nursing homes tend to be selective in accepting patients, choosing those with care requirements that are at a level that permits them to make a (reasonable) profit and compensates them for the difficulties that certain types of patients create. In areas of the country where compensation is adequate in the eyes of the nursing home operators, nursing homes accept even the most difficult patients. In the east, where compensation is lower, nursing homes readily accept low-care, low-cost, low-difficulty patients and, by their actions, leave the balance in the hospital where the cost of maintenance is higher and the normal and intended operations of the hospital are disrupted.

Home care. Each of the hospitals has developed arrangements or affiliations for providing visiting-nurse and home-health services to the community. These services appear, however, to vary quite substantially in their scope and achievements. In five of the hospitals, the home-care nursing services are provided by employees of the hospital. In the balance of the institutions, the services are rendered by local Visiting Nurse Associations (VNAs) or their equivalent private or governmental agencies.

At first glance, one is apt to identify ownership by the hospital as of primary importance. However, there are other indications that it is not critical, for very satisfactory relationships and high quality services are provided under other arrangements. What is critical is (1) the doctors' knowledge of the range of services offered and their confidence in the quality of the work performed and (2) the extent to which postdischarge planning for the individual patient is facilitated by ready access to the home-care-nursing personnel.

In hospitals in which home-care nursing is most extensively used, employees of the hospital's home care department or the VNA have offices in the hospital and easy access to all areas and jointly plan postdischarge care with the doctors, floor nurses, the patient, and the patient's family. In these situations, the person-to-person contacts and the ease with which arrangements can be made are both considered important.

At times, reimbursement provisions create a problem. Thus, it is of interest that one hospital director noted that a couple of hospitals in his area have made an agreement with Blue Cross whereby the hospital will release patients one or two days earlier than normal and then provide necessary services to these patients at home (including many diagnostic and therapeutic exams) through visiting-nurse services. The nurses make their rounds in well-equipped vans, accompanied by electrocardiogram (EKG) technicians or other types of trained specialists. This progam has proved to be cost effective and has also improved bed availability.

The Kaiser-Permanente representatives we interviewed indicated that the concept of controlling the home-health care program is strongly supported in that organization as well. The administrative director of one division stated, ". . . while we used to have much longer obstetrical stays, we try now to get them out on the second day, as soon as the mother and child are capable. But we do have the home-health people make one nursing call to be sure that the baby hasn't developed jaundice, etc., to see that the mother's taking care of the baby satisfactorily, and that the mother is o.k." In most areas, however, home health services have not approached their full potential. It is our impression that efforts expended in this pursuit could be quite productive.

III

Making the Hospital an Efficient Instrument Through Responsive Ancillary and Other Hospital-based Services

Doctors and patients in a modern hospital are so dependent upon the services provided by hospital-based departments that the responsiveness of these departments to doctors' requirements — measured in terms of range of services, extent of coverage, and speed of response — significantly affects a hospital's quality of care, the length of stay of its patients and its rate of occupancy. Some evidence of this has already been provided by the discussion (particularly of off-peak utilization) in the preceding section. The influence of ancillary departments is, however, pervasive — affecting all patients and doctors regardless of which days of the week are involved.

In this chapter, comments will be made on a variety of topics (the asterisked topics are covered more fully than the others):

- Radiology services*
- Laboratory services*
- Outpatient services
- Preadmission testing*
- Operating rooms*
- Physical therapy
- Patient transport
- Consultant services

While this section concerns primarily the role of the hospital and hospital-based physicians in providing ancillary services, attention will also be directed to the disparity among individual attending physicians in their ability to make efficient use of the services that are available and the efforts they make to do so. Comments on this point were made with great frequency, not only by the service-providing departments but also by attending physicians and nursing directors. This topic will be covered to a greater degree in Chapter IV.

RADIOLOGY SERVICES

The preceding introductory comments can be underlined with respect to radiology for, of all the ancillary services, those rendered by this department have the greatest impact on a hospital's ability to achieve a low length of stay.

Both turnaround time and hours of availability are important — the former primarily because of its effect on virtually all patients and the latter because of its greater impact on a smaller but still significant number of patients. This is confirmed by Perry and Baum,* who in their discussion of radiology department performance, state that delays in handling diagnostic reports contribute directly to increased patient-care costs and to length of stay. They refer, in fact, to a 1971 study by Gertman and Becker in which it was found that, at that time, "approximately sixteen percent of the inappropriate** days of hospital stay were caused by delayed radiological reports."

There are a number of reasons why radiological availability and turnaround time have an important impact on a patient's rate of progress:

1. Because radiological procedures usually constitute key elements of the diagnostic process, treatment (usually by surgery) and recovery cannot begin until they have been completed. Thus, the progress of patients not diagnosed prior to admission can be seriously affected.
2. Because the radiological process is complex — even when the x-ray it-

---

* Perry and Baum, "Resource Allocation and Scheduling for a Radiology Dept." in *Cost Control in Hospitals*, by Griffith, et al., (Ann Arbor: Health Administration Press, 1976), p. 230.

** A day was defined as "inappropriate" if the major reason for that day's stay was not directly related to patient diagnosis or treatment.

self is simple — the opportunities for delaying any or all patients are considerable. The process involves (1) ordering the test by the physician, (2) scheduling the test, (3) patient transportation and patient management while awaiting an available room, (4) taking the actual x-ray, (5) patient return, (6) interpretation by the radiologist, (7) typing of the report by x-ray department typists, (8) delivery of the report to the nursing station, (9) placement of the report on the patient's chart, (10) study of the report by the physician and, if needed, (11) consultation with the radiologist by the physician. These well-known facts are recited because the waiting or "inactive time" involved between these steps often far exceeds the "active time" spent in carrying them out and since many departments and individuals are involved, both inter- and intradepartmental procedures must be managed effectively for efficient performance.

3. Because of their personal participation in performing special procedures, interpreting x-rays, and consulting with physicians, the availability and working habits of radiologists are critical. Radiological technicians cannot perform these functions and emergency room physicians only preliminarily interpret films in the absence of the radiologists.

AVAILABILITY OF SERVICE

Tables III-1 and 2 display the hours of service offered at the various hospitals included in the study. In-house coverage is relatively standard in most hospitals on weekdays (generally 8:30 A.M.–5:00 P.M.) and Saturday (8:00 A.M.–12:00 noon). During off-hours, the schedules provide that routine x-rays will be taken by radiological technicians and temporarily interpreted by attending and emergency room physicians (pending subsequent official interpretation by a radiologist) unless the requirements of the particular case need the services of an on-call radiologist. Special procedures are not available during off-hours except on an emergency, on-call basis.

In practice, most radiologists are more than willing to remain in the department past the normal closing time in order to finish the day's work or to accommodate a specific request from an attending physician. They also are uniformly available during off-hours for emergencies, if requested by an attending physician. The basic question, however, remains as to whether this type of coverage is sufficient.

In nearly every institution, most or all of the attending physicians we interviewed described a causal relationship between the hours when radiologists are available in-house for special procedures and consultations

TABLE III-1

In-House Radiologist Availability

Monday — Friday

Radiologist Arrival Time

At 7 A.M.	4 Hospitals
At 7:30 A.M.	2 Hospitals
At 8 A.M. or later	8 Hospitals
Information not available	1 Hospital

Radiologist Departure Time

At 4:30 P.M.	2 Hospitals
Between 5:00 and 5:30 P.M.	6 Hospitals
Between 6:00 and 7:00 P.M.	5 Hospitals
At 8 P.M. or later	2 Hospitals

Saturday

Arrival Time

Before 8 A.M.	1 Hospital
At 8 A.M.	13 Hospitals
At 8:30 A.M.	1 Hospital

Departure Time

"As early as possible"	2 Hospitals
Before Noon	1 Hospital
Between 12 and 12:30 P.M.	8 Hospitals
At 4 P.M.	1 Hospital
At 6 P.M.	1 Hospital
Information not specified	2 Hospitals

Sunday and Holidays

On call (or come in to clean up)	10 Hospitals
8 A.M.-12 noon	1 Hospital
9 A.M.-12 noon	1 Hospital
8 A.M.-4 P.M.	1 Hospital
8 A.M.-10 P.M.	1 Hospital
10 A.M.-6 P.M.	1 Hospital

TABLE III–2

EXAMPLES OF TECHNICAL STAFF COVERAGE
RADIOLOGY AND LABORATORY DEPARTMENTS

All hospitals provide around-the-clock coverage for emergency procedures in both the radiology and laboratory departments. Identified below are examples of extended coverage for elective procedures.

RADIOLOGY

MONDAY — FRIDAY

Day Shift Staff Reports to Work At:

6:30 A.M.	3 Hospitals
7:00 A.M.	3 Hospitals
7:30 A.M. or later	7 Hospitals
Information not specified	2 Hospitals

WEEKENDS

Saturday

Full coverage 8 A.M. – 4:30 P.M.	2 Hospitals
Full coverage, Saturday morning only	12 Hospitals
Information not specified	1 Hospital

Sunday

No elective coverage specified	14 Hospitals
Information not specified	1 Hospital

LABORATORY

MONDAY – FRIDAY

Day Shift Reports to Work At:

5 A.M.	3 Hospitals
5:30 A.M.	1 Hospital
6 A.M.	1 Hospital
6:30–6:45 A.M.	2 Hospitals
7 A.M. or later	6 Hospitals
Information not specified	2 Hospitals

(One institution provides full staffing until 11 P.M.)

WEEKENDS

No significant findings

TABLE III–3

In–House Pathology Availability

Monday — Friday

Pathologist Arrival Time

Before 7 A.M.	1 Hospital
Betweeen 7 and 8 A.M.	10 Hospitals
Between 8 and 9 A.M.	2 Hospitals
Information not available	2 Hospitals

Pathologist Departure Time

At 5 P.M.	5 Hospitals
Between 5 and 6 P.M.	3 Hospitals
Between 6 and 7 P.M.	2 Hospitals
Information not specified	5 Hospitals

Saturday

Arrival Time

Before 7 A.M.	1 Hospital
Between 7 and 8 A.M.	9 Hospitals
Not specified	5 Hospitals

Departure Time

12 noon or earlier	5 Hospitals
Between 12 and 2 P.M.	4 Hospitals
Between 4 and 5 P.M.	2 Hospitals
Not specified	4 Hospitals

Sunday and Holidays

Two hospitals have in–house coverage from 8 A.M. to 12 noon. Others have on call pathologists.

---

and the physicians' ability to reach judgments quickly about the future course of a patient's care. Where radiologists are least available, lack of coverage is frequently described not only as being an operational problem that slows patient care, but also as a source of irritation between the attending physicians and radiologists. Where in-house radiologist coverage is the most extensive, the attending physicians have little but praise for the radiology departments. Few, if any, of the physicians with whom we spoke suggested that the radiologists should significantly increase their individual hours of availability. Rather they suggested that coverage could be expanded through staggered hours.

At two hospitals, coverage that substantially exceeds the general pattern is provided. There the hospitals and radiologists provide full in-house radiological coverage from 8:00 A.M. to 10:00 P.M. and 8:00 A.M. to 6:00 P.M., seven days a week. In one hospital, coverage is provided exclusively by members of the regular full-time staff on a rotating basis while at the second institution, permanent, part-time radiologists provide coverage after 6:00 P.M. and on weekends. Both the radiologists and the attending physicians at these institutions said the effects of this extended coverage are important.

1. It extends the period during which emergency and other inpatients can receive diagnostic services, and it speeds their process of treatment by making the results available to the attending physicians more rapidly on both weekdays and weekends.
2. It improves the availability and speed of radiologic service and interpretation of at least certain procedures required by emergency room patients.
3. It provides more convenient hours for some PAT patients and outpatients and simultaneously removes that load from the radiology department's busiest hours.
4. It makes therapeutic treatments available at times that some patients find more suitable.
5. It increases the number of tests that can be made with a given number of x-ray rooms and complement of equipment, and
6. It encourages weekend occupancy by making it more productive for doctors and patients to use the hospital.

We would not profess, on the basis of our study, to know how the question of coverage should be resolved. However, we feel that the examples provided by two hospitals that have successfully extended radiological hours and the results that they have achieved are important to hospitals whose bed situation and other objectives require that the intensity of off-hours or weekend operations be increased.

RESPONSE TIME

It is our impression that speed of response is far more closely correlated with radiologist behavior, managerial competence, staffing patterns and skills, and information-producing and delivery procedures than with the sophistication of radiological equipment and the adequacy of the space allocated to the department. No doubt modern, reliable equipment and adequate space are important for a variety of purposes, but we observed a number of institutions that, in spite of disadvantages, respond impressively to physicians' requests for service.

This conclusion is not surprising in view of the facts that (1) the waiting or inactive time often exceeds the active time spent in carrying out the radiological process; and (2) the greatest opportunity to improve response time, in most instances, lies in reducing the amount of time in which little or nothing is happening. To a certain extent, this requires looking at the eleven-step process described on page 43 as an entire system, as few, if any, of the hospitals seem to have done; to a greater extent, the individual delays can be attacked separately, as has been the normal procedure.

Some of the more effective steps taken to improve the response time for all or selected procedures are briefly described below:

1. *Priorities* — All hospitals have schedules that attempt to accommodate the various categories of patients during different periods of the day but permit adjustments for unscheduled requirements. The usual order of priorities is, as might be expected: (a) present inpatients, requiring diagnostic x-rays to permit treatment to proceed; (b) scheduled inpatients, requiring x-rays to complete preadmission testing (or the equivalent that is given on arrival); and (c) outpatients. Critical and urgent patients are given priority over those in better condition.

   The interesting differences among hospitals is their practice with respect to outpatient business. Most hospitals consider outpatient x-ray work a supplement to inpatient hospital service and attempt to schedule it when the department will not be busy with inpatient work. Often, however, they find that such a position is difficult to sustain under competitive conditions. Some hospitals have, therefore, increased their staff and equipment to handle outpatients on favorable terms, but others are attempting to meet the situation with less-than-complete success insofar as inpatient progress is concerned. This is one of the factors leading several hospitals to reexamine their basic attitude toward outpatient work — as will be discussed subsequently in this section.

   The assignment of priorities to special procedures provides a somewhat more difficult problem, particularly when they are lengthy and complex and must be carried out by the radiologists themselves in only one or two rooms. Nevertheless, all hospitals make efforts to give top priority to special procedures in the morning and a high priority to them throughout the day. In all but one hospital, inpatients are given priority over outpatients for such procedures. Interestingly, in that particular hospital outpatients are given priority on the grounds that they have less flexibility in their personal schedules and, therefore, are less likely to tolerate delays.

2. *Starting times* — Most hospitals attempt to provide x-ray service to inpatients as early in the day as is practical because, in part, the patients are already available and, in part, because this may enable the radiology department to provide attending physicians with their reports during their morning rounds. However, hospitals' definitions of "as early as is practical" differ.

In some hospitals, the technical staff (and in two cases, the departmentally dedicated transport staff) begin their work at staggered times as early as 7:00 A.M. Regular procedures are carried out by x-ray technicians upon the patient's arrival in the radiology department, with the films thus becoming available for interpretation by the radiologists at an early hour. In addition, patients requiring special procedures are brought to the radiology department, ready for the radiologist(s) to begin the procedures immediately upon their arrival between 7:30 A.M. and 8:00 A.M., i.e., an hour earlier than in most other institutions. Both regular and special procedures are thus completed earlier in the day, and the reports are dictated and transcribed and made available to doctors more quickly. Patients are returned to their rooms earlier and have a greater likelihood of being available for other types of diagnostic or therapeutic activities (including meals) on that day. In addition, the x-ray rooms become available for more of the same or other types of procedures. Institutions that use this schedule have not increased the total hours worked by their technical staff but rather have redistributed them over a greater portion of the day.

3. *PAT patients*–Some hospitals, particularly those with more limited preadmission testing, make special provision to handle newly admitted patients by providing especially effective service in the late afternoon.

4. *Transport* — The general issues relating to patient transportation are discussed on page 71. At this point, it is of interest to note that five hospitals had dedicated transport personnel in their radiology departments. While some problems were experienced with late arrivals even with dedicated transport personnel, these were considered to be of lesser proportions than had previously been encountered. But, with or without dedicated personnel, the usual situation seems

to be to require that patients wait in halls or waiting rooms in order to minimize unused procedure-room time.

5. *Transcription* — A number of interesting efforts are being made to improve the speed of transcription. Most, but not all, hospitals recognize the crucial importance of this function and are staffing this position with a more adequate number of more highly skilled and trained transcriptionists than in the past. They also are making limited but effective use of preprogrammed, automatic typewriters, especially on films with negative results. Principally, however, they are adjusting staffing hours to match workload. They are, for example:
   a. Staggering the starting times of transcriptionists in the morning so that staffing more closely coincides with the workload (which tends to be heavier later in the day).
   b. Hiring part-time transcriptionists for evening and weekend shifts who are responsible for (1) completing all outstanding reports for the day, (2) taking the typed reports to the nursing units, and (3) personally placing them on the patient charts.
   c. Permitting daytime transcriptionists to remain, at overtime pay, until all reports are completed.

6. *Delivery* — The delivery of the finished reports to the nursing units and their placement on the patients' charts are often the source of substantial delays, out of all proportion to the simplicity of the tasks involved, not only during evenings and weekends, when this might be expected, but also during regular weekday hours. The most radical and, in many respects, the most effective and psychologically satisfying solution encountered is for the transcriptionists themselves to place the reports on the charts, available for the doctors' use. In other hospitals, other radiology department employees — especially, dedicated transport personnel — are also used for this purpose. Placement on the chart is emphasized in quite a few hospitals because of the length of time that frequently elapses between delivery of the reports to the nursing unit and their availability on patients' charts when nursing department clerks must be relied on to perform the placement function.

Managing the Department

One important question that emerged concerns a specific managerial question: "Who is managing the radiology department?" In a sense, the question deals in a small area with a matter that concerns the hospital as a whole. However, in this instance, the problem is particularly acute, for very little of the work of the department can proceed without the personal participation at key points of radiologists who do not report organizationally to the department manager. At the same time, it is a department of persons with diverse skills who are dependent to a substantial degree on the work of those who precede them in the process and who report in all medical respects, de facto, to the radiologists. It is a situation with few parallels in business or elsewhere.

It is our impression — although we would be hard put to prove it — that the effectiveness of many radiology departments, as measured in terms of response, is significantly affected by:

1. the quality and attitudes of the radiologists,
2. the strength and role of the department manager,
3. the quality of his relationship with the radiologists, and
4. the radiologists' understanding and acceptance of their department's role as a key element in a patient's overall progress rather than as an essentially self-contained unit rendering important medical services.

It is clear that radiologists, because of their role and prestige, have to support and work constructively with the managerial efforts of the department manager. At least as important, they have to subordinate whatever personal instincts they may have that conflict with the essentially "production line" nature of the department's role — by being available on schedule, promptly dictating reports, observing departmental routines, and otherwise setting a good personal example. It is probably true that, in a number of hospitals, the success of improvement efforts will depend to an important degree on changes in the radiologists' pattern of work and the greater acceptance of their overall role as part of a system.

LABORATORY SERVICES

A great deal of similarity exists among the laboratories we visited. While brands of equipment vary, most are at essentially similar levels of automation. (For example, all but one hospital has automated equipment for multi-phasic screening in chemistry — SMA-12, SMAC, etc.) There is also a good deal of consistency in what is done in–house and what is sent to outside laboratories. The laboratories are uniformly well regarded by the medical staff for the quality of their work. And, finally, there is recognition by pathologists and attending physicians alike that patient progress is related to the availability and speed of service that the laboratory provides.

RESPONSE TIME AND HOURS OF SERVICE

Response time, from a doctor's point of view, can be defined as the total time that elapses between a physician's order for a test and the availability of the test results to him. As such, laboratory response time has three components:

1. the hours and days during which laboratory services are available for tests and consultations,
2. the length of time that the laboratory requires to perform the test and record the test results, and
3. the efficiency with which test requests and specimens are collected and test results are delivered and placed on the patients' charts.

From the standpoint of rate of occupancy and length of stay, the first and last of the three components are important. This is reflected in the fact that, in spite of the present level of performance, a number of doctors expressed a desire for greater coverage for tests and consultations and faster turnaround times for test results.

Tables III-2 (p. 45) and III-3 contain information about the basic hours of service provided by the laboratories at the hospitals we visited. It shows that (1) all hospitals provide services for critical patients on an emergency basis 24 hours a day, seven days a week, but (2) the hours and days during which work is carried out for noncritical patients vary considerably. By and large, the hours shown as available for routine work represent the hours that the technicians are available. The pathologists normally are present to carry out the special tests that they perform, to support physicians during operations involving biopsies, to consult with technicians with respect to difficult tests and interpretations, and otherwise to participate in departmental activities during somewhat more limited periods. Pathologists usually are available for consultations with physicians during their normal periods of work and are on call for emergency assistance at other times.

Several items are worthy of note:

1. The laboratory tends to differ from the radiology department in that (1) it presently provides services to noncritical patients over a longer period of time; (2) its work involves a process that usually is shorter and less complex, requires fewer people, and does not involve moving the patient; and (3) most of its tests are carried out by a technician and are interpreted by the attending physician, without the participation of a pathologist.
2. Because of the nature of the process and the extent of the patholo-

gists' participation, an extension of hours usually involves only the addition of technician hours (that are paid for by the hospital, since technicians are hospital employees). For the vast majority of the laboratory's work, decisions about extended hours or staggered hours tend, therefore, to be based primarily on considerations of hospital efficiency with which the pathologists normally find little fault.

Laboratories use two basic approaches in providing increased coverage with the same volume of work.

1. They distribute the same total departmental hours over a greater portion of the day by staggering the hours of work of selected employees at the start and close of the day.
2. They redistribute their staff over days of the week.

These approaches will be noted in the examples of extended coverage that are described below.

One of the more effective ways of improving response times that we encountered is achieved by advancing blood collection times in the morning to a point where the test results are on the chart by the time most doctors make their morning rounds. In at least three hospitals, test results for certain classifications of patients (newborns, ICU, CCU, and certain preoperative patients) are on the charts by 9:00 A.M. because phlebotomists or other laboratory personnel draw blood samples as early as 5:00 A.M. Test results for other patients are, as a consequence, also available at an earlier hour than would otherwise be the case. Two institutions stagger their personnel in order to cover the early morning hours, while the third hospital hires moonlighters, who hold full-time jobs elsewhere.*

At an additional three hospitals, laboratory personnel begin gathering samples at 5:30 or 6:00 A.M. None of these six institutions reports problems with patients concerning the early hour at which specimens are drawn, and each reports very favorable reactions from doctors and improved laboratory efficiency.

The incoming patient without preadmission testing, who is admitted in the afternoon, is another classification of patient whose length of stay can easily be increased by a whole day in the absence of efficient laboratory work, sometimes through extended hours. To make the test results on the

---

* The moonlighters are guaranteed payment for a minimum of two hours daily. If they complete their rounds more quickly, they still receive the minimum payment but may leave.

patients' charts available not later than the first thing the following day, several hospitals combine (1) immediate blood collection procedures in which blood samples of newly admitted patients are collected before the patients proceed to their rooms, (2) a priority system in the laboratory, and (3) adequate regular or flexible hours of work in the afternoon or evening.

As Table III-3 indicates, some hospitals provide substantial coverage for nonemergency laboratory tests on weekday evenings and on Saturdays and Sundays. All hospitals agree that this affects patients who are already in the hospital, patients arriving later in the day than those described in the preceding paragraph, and — of substantial importance — those who would be admitted if the service were available. They differ, however, in their estimates of the extent of the impact on their institutions and even about how one can reasonably determine it in view of the complexity of the factors at work. In the several institutions providing substantial Saturday and Sunday services, it is believed that the ready availability of diagnostic tests keep those days from being essentially custodial days for many patients and, because these services are available, physicians are more inclined to admit patients and aggressively use the hospital on weekends. These hospitals intend to continue the extended coverage, being satisfied on the basis of logic and general observation rather than a detailed analysis of service implications, costs, and revenues.

In the situation in which a hospital finds it desirable or essential to operate with a high weekend census and a low length of stay in order to accommodate its patients and doctors, it must depend upon the availability of extensive laboratory services to all patients during expanded service hours. The fact that in some hospitals a wide range of laboratory services is available to all patients beyond normal periods is, thus, of importance. Pathologists in several other institutions said they were quite willing to extend their departmental hours to meet doctor requirements.

Much of the foregoing discussion deals with the manner in which the laboratory can support doctors' efforts by making services available outside normal hours. It deals with rather obvious groups of patients — those needing early morning results, those arriving in mid-to-late afternoon, and those admitted in the evening and on weekends (particularly Sundays).

We hoped to find hospitals that had studied one of the more subtle aspects of the problem — the interrelationship of physician behavior, laboratory staffing, and optimum test-response time. This is a particularly acute problem where attending physicians spend relatively limited portions of the day at the hospital. If they do not receive test results during their rounds, a patient's diagnosis, treatment — and even recovery — can be delayed by as much as a day. Nearly all the pathologists indicate that they feel pressure from the attending physicians for more rapid turnaround time on laboratory test results. This pressure exists not only in hospitals with comparatively long turnaround times, but also in those that respond most quickly. However, no institution had studied precisely when physicians order tests and when test results would best assist doctors in determining a patient's future course of treatment. Studies, including the one by Perry and Baum (op. cit.), have shown that as many as 75 percent of physician visits to hospitalized patients occur between the hours of 8:00 A.M. and 12 noon and that it is highly probable that laboratory or diagnostic radiology reports will not be seen or used by the physician until the following day if those results are not available prior to noon. However, 8 A.M. to 12 noon is itself a rather lengthy period, particularly because the results of many laboratory tests tend to become available in the later part of that period. On that basis, one might conclude that at best, laboratory staffing patterns are designed only to approximate the flow of demand and/or that a faster response with test results might reap greater benefits. At worst, it is possible that laboratory staffing is designed primarily for the convenience of the laboratory and may be causing dysfunctions in the hospital system as a whole — dysfunctions that can be substantially lessened by more flexible staffing patterns. Both the facts and the solution could be of considerable interest and value.

AVAILABILITY FOR CONSULTATION

In most instances, physicians interpret test results directly from data placed on the patient's chart; interpretative reports normally are prepared only for special tests whose meanings are not immediately clear. Consultations with pathologists are relatively infrequent, although important when they occur.

We were told at two institutions that the ready accessibility of pathologists for consultations has made a noticeable difference in the speed of patient care. While some pathologists emphasize their efforts to be accessible to attending physicians, we did not encounter any institution in which pathologists are routinely available for consultations late in the evening. In only one case are they available for nonemergency patients after noon on Saturday, even though they are on call for emergencies during those times.

OPERATING ROOM SUPPORT

An important aspect of a pathologist's work involves his support of surgeons who are performing procedures in which immediate analysis of the patient's condition (e.g., the presence of cancerous cells) is required to determine how to continue the operation. In this regard the availability of pathologists does not seem to be a limiting factor.

TEST-PROCESSING TIME

Test-processing time — the second of the components of response time — did not emerge as a problem of significant proportions in the hospitals visited. Undoubtedly, a detailed analysis of the procedures and operations of several laboratories would show variations in productivity and opportunities for improvement in processing time. However, the important conclusion from the perspective of this study is that such improvement would not significantly affect length of stay and rate of occupancy. On the other hand, when test results are so delayed that doctors frequently must phone the laboratory, the resultant disruption reduces the productivity of the laboratory and does delay the process of patient care.

COLLECTION AND COMMUNICATION SYSTEMS

The foregoing discussion of hours of service adequately covers the points we wish to make relative to specimen collection. We'd like now to comment on the various systems of communicating test requisitions and results.

Most hospitals use some form of manual or pneumatic system for this purpose. In the manual systems, multi-part laboratory requisition forms are completed on the nursing unit and collected by mail, transport, or laboratory personnel — depending on the institution and the time of day. Where pneumatic systems exist, they usually are used to send test requisitions to the laboratory.

However, we found that even though they are available, pneumatic systems are not always used, either because nurses do not find the location of the tubes convenient or because of a lack of confidence in the system's reliability. In all systems, once tests have been completed, the results are manually transported or sent through the pneumatic tube back to the unit.

There does not appear to be a correlation between major differences in average turnaround time and whether a manual or pneumatic tube system is used for the transmission of requisitions and results. Rather, differences seem to vary primarily in relation to (1) the frequency of pick-up and delivery to the nursing units and (2) whether laboratory personnel or nursing unit clerks are responsible for placing test results on the patient's chart.

Laboratory computer systems appear to make a difference, a finding based on observations made during this study and another investigation we have made that concerns the desirability of acquiring a laboratory computer. Test requisitions transmitted by wire from nursing units permit the laboratory to start testing immediately after the specimen is drawn. However, while there are certain advantages to be gained from using wire transmission for all test requests, there also are costs and disadvantages that tend to limit their use severely. Thus, they tend to be used in situations where the need for speed is greatest (e.g., in the ICU, CCU, and ER) and the specimen is to be drawn immediately — rather than at a later time, as is very often the case.

Wire transmission of test results has a distinct advantage in terms of speed. As soon as they are completed, test results can appear on a CRT display panel at the nursing unit upon the doctor's request. Hard copy results are recorded on the patient's chart later on, but the time required to get them there does not affect the patient's progress.**

TESTS PER ADMISSION

In spite of the general similarity of their laboratory equipment, there seem to be substantial differences among the hospitals visited in the number of laboratory tests performed per admission. The reasons for and the extent of these differences are not clear. The extent is clouded by differences in counting procedures and definitions that make statistical comparisons across state lines hazardous. The reasons include not only differences in the degree to which outside laboratories are used, but also the general attitude of the medical staff toward the value of laboratory test data and the pathologists' efforts to educate physicians in its use.

It is obvious that excessive testing is unduly expensive and can adversely affect length of stay. It is equally clear that testing can have a beneficial effect through sharpened diagnosis and more effective treatment. In this respect, the amount of testing done involves medical judgments that are beyond the level of competence of this study. However, several points of general interest can be made:

1. Hospitals whose medical audit and utilization review program are establishing standard or suggested treatment patterns are now con-

---

** It may be of interest that two of the hospitals visited found that, no matter what the computer's other merits were, (a) the number and cost of hired computer specialists exceeded the number and cost of eliminated clerical positions, and (b) technical staffs were not affected.

cerning themselves with the types of tests to be given and sometimes with their frequency.

2. As part of cost control efforts being carried out internally on a voluntary basis or imposed externally by a reimbursing or other agency, the numbers and types of tests are being more carefully scrutinized than in the past.

3. Continuing reductions in length of stay may be causing a reduction in the number of laboratory tests.

Whatever the reasons, there is some feeling that, after a long period of slow, consistent increases, the number of tests per patient may be leveling off or slightly declining.

THE DESIRABILITY OF PROVIDING OUTPATIENT SERVICES

All of the hospitals provide outpatient laboratory and radiological services to two classes of patients:

1. Those scheduled to be admitted as inpatients who are obtaining preadmission tests, and

2. others, not scheduled for admission, referred by doctors for a variety of diagnostic purposes.

The first category of patients is of substantial importance. Most hospitals credit PAT with important reductions in length of stay and, therefore, make special efforts to make their facilities available at hours that are convenient for those purposes.

The second category of patients appears to be more controversial, with a surprising number of hospitals expressing an ambivalent or discouraged attitude about the desirability of outpatient work. In fact, some have taken steps to reduce the volume of outpatients and to be more selective in the tests performed. Others are planning to implement such policies through future construction and operational decisions.

The reasons are mainly physical and economic. In hospitals with inadequate space, the consensus is that outpatient services interfere with inpatient care. Even where space is adequate, conflicts exist in the timing of inpatient and outpatient tests — a troublesome situation unless staff and equipment are adequate to handle both. More frequently than hospitals would like, this situation can result in prolonging patient stays.

Increased competition and pricing are also seen by some hospitals as a source of present and future problems. They cite not only the inherently lower cost structure of laboratories located in doctors' offices and commercial settings, but also the present and potential restrictions on prices established by regulatory and reimbursing agencies.

On the positive side, some hospitals find that outpatient tests are financially attractive and that they make good use of staff, equipment, and space. They note the benefits derived from adding outpatient volume to inpatient requirements on tests utilizing expensive equipment. They point to the more extended hours on both weekdays and weekends when their services are available. They cite greater assurance of quality over a wide range of tests they offer. Finally, they believe that with effort and ingenuity and policies that give priority to inpatients, potential problems can be minimized to a point where a net benefit exists.

In some cities, hospitals seek to provide outpatient services outside of the hospital, primarily in doctors' office buildings. In other areas, the hospital's own doctors are encouraged and permitted to develop their own outpatient facilities (a practice prohibited by other hospitals). Another alternative which we did not encounter, but which we can visualize, would be that in which a hospital chooses to be selective in the outpatient services it renders by performing the more specialized tests, especially those requiring expensive skills and equipment, and/or by covering those periods of the day and week when commercial facilities are closed — and by charging premium prices for those services, just as the emergency room now does in its role of "temporary doctor."

PREADMISSION TESTING

Among the more obvious and directly beneficial ways of minimizing the stay of elective patients is the completion of all or nearly all of the diagnostic aspects of the patient's care prior to admission. Preadmission testing (PAT) programs, designed to accomplish this objective, exist in nearly all of the institutions visited. However, the degree of emphasis placed on the program, the scope of available services, and the frequency with which it is employed vary considerably. Institutions using PAT most actively are convinced that the program has a marked positive effect on their hospital's length of stay and they have statistical information that appears to substantiate this claim. In fact, physicians in one hospital indicate that demands made by anesthesiologists to see laboratory results well in advance of surgery contributes to the use of PAT, speeds laboratory turnaround time, and significantly reduces the number of patients whose surgery is cancelled just prior to surgery because of suddenly-found medical contraindications.

The keys to a successful PAT program appear to be the following:

1. an institutional commitment to the program that includes a willingness to commit staffing and resources necessary for an effective program,
2. services that are readily available to patients at convenient times and locations and that provide the information needed by physicians in a timely manner, and
3. a medical staff that understands the importance of the program (including its potential impact on bed availability) and encourages or directs their patients to use it.

Interesting aspects of the PAT programs in the hospitals we visited are noted in this chapter.

PAT STAFF

Staffing for PAT programs varies dramatically. In several institutions, no particular person coordinates the program. Instead, the admitting office and individual physicians are responsible for scheduling tests and compiling results. Elsewhere, the PAT program is coordinated by from 0.5 to 2.5 full-time equivalent specialized clerks or RNs. Although many hospitals use RNs because registered nurses can accept physician orders over the phone, at least one program appears to be highly successful without RNs on the staff. However, in that hospital, a great deal of effort has gone into the development and distribution of preprinted PAT requisition forms that physicians can quickly complete in their offices.

PERIOD OF VALIDITY OF PAT WORK

A drawback to PAT mentioned in several hospitals is that the cancellation of a patient's admission due to a lack of beds requires that much of the PAT work must be repeated before the patient is admitted at a later date. This is costly for the hospital and inconvenient for the patient. If bed availability is chronically poor, this can develop into a vicious cycle for, as more patients are cancelled, physicians will use PAT less frequently, choosing instead to admit patients for immediate presurgical, diagnostic testing. In turn, this reduces overall bed availability even further unless very efficient postadmission testing procedures (sometimes known as "early day testing," or EDT) are employed, and increases the possibility that additional PAT patients will be cancelled.

The major assumption underlying this problem is that PAT results are valid for such a limited period of time that cancellation of the original admission date almost automatically requires that the laboratory, and often the EKG portions of the PAT program, be repeated. In most of the hospitals we visited, laboratory results are considered useful for not more than 48 or 72 hours. However, in several hospitals, test results are considered valid for more than seven days (with a maximum observed limit of fourteen days). In these cases either no tests are repeated or only those where the patient exhibited a marginal condition. Since physicians and employees at institutions with longer periods of validity express satisfaction with and no concern about the practice in their hospitals, medical staffs at other hospitals may find it desirable to review their more restrictive policies.

Extension of the validity period for PAT work also encourages the program's use by giving patients greater flexibility in choosing when they will undergo tests. It also reduces the pressure to return the results of PAT tests immediately. If a patient is not to be admitted for several days, ancillary departments can handle tests in a more routine manner.

PHYSICIAN AND PATIENT CONVENIENCE

In order to encourage the use of PAT, at least three hospitals make the necessary services available in the evenings and on Saturdays. This significantly increases use of PAT by individuals who have daytime jobs. While ancillary departments must be adequately staffed during these times, the volume of work has more than justified the modest increase in man-hours. More important, by moving PAT work to evenings and Saturdays, hospitals decrease the work load of ancillary departments during other, traditionally busier periods.

Two hospitals permit at least a portion of PAT work to be performed outside the hospital by approved, licensed laboratories. Despite a number of possible advantages to the patient and doctor, this approach has received limited acceptance. Hospitals resist largely on the basis of quality concerns, and require that specific tests be made by the hospital laboratory. And the reimbursement systems either consider such out-of-hospital tests to be nonreimbursable or reimbursable to a limited, inadequate maximum. Obviously there are numerous issues to be considered. But, assuming that quality concerns can be satisfied by inspection procedures or other means, one could visualize a situation in which hospitals might attempt to influence regulatory and reimbursing agencies, at least in instances where distance or other problems made PAT excessively inconvenient for certain classes of patients.

In most hospitals with successful PAT programs, convenient parking is provided for PAT patients, and access to the necessary ancillary services and movement between them are made as easy and free of red tape as is practical. Administrators frequently indicate that easy access to PAT services is a major contributor to the success of the program in view of the physical condition of some patients and the devastating effect that unfavorable reactions of patients can have on the future actions of their doctors.

EFFICIENT DAY-OF-ADMISSION TESTING AS AN ALTERNATIVE TO PAT

Three hospitals have chosen not to use PAT procedures or have limited them severely, putting their efforts instead into impressively efficient testing, with rapid turnaround times, once the patient has been admitted to the hospital (again, EDT programs). In one hospital, the number of cancelled admissions is too great. In a second, the inconvenience and loss of time is too burdensome for rural patients. In the third hospital, extended ancillary department hours, plus efficiency, have resulted in better service for all those admitted.

These hospitals acknowledge that they cannot prevent the admission of elective patients whose postadmission tests reveal conditions that must be treated before surgery can take place. In these instances, they usually discharge and readmit the patient, finding that, in their circumstances, the resultant inconveniences are insufficient to make them move toward PAT.

OPERATING ROOMS

In a typical hospital, more than half of all patients undergo a surgical procedure during the course of their hospitalization. Accordingly, the availability of adequate operating time critically affects the flow of patients, the length of their stay, and the rate of occupancy of the institution. In important ways, it affects the ability of a surgeon and his elective patient to plan and schedule admission to the hospital and thus is both a convenience and a competitive factor.

AVAILABILITY OF OPERATING ROOM TIME

Requirements for operating time per bed/day are increasing. Many of those interviewed expect these requirements to become still greater because of:

1. reductions in overall length of stay and the resulting increase in the number of surgical admissions per bed/year,
2. changes in surgical practices resulting in an increase in the number

of more complex and time-consuming procedures performed, and
3. increased outpatient surgery.

Some hospitals already have taken steps such as establishing dedicated ambulatory surgery facilities directed at preventing operating room bottlenecks. Other institutions, while attempting primarily to reduce operating room and overall hospital costs, see this "streamlining" as a secondary objective.

STRATEGIC CONSIDERATIONS

As an important element of overall hospital strategy, hospitals are re-examining the trade-off of costs and benefits of operating time in terms of the overall impact on operating rooms, bed occupancy, and doctor-patient relations. Not surprisingly, this leads different hospitals to reach different conclusions to fit their specific circumstances. It is perhaps surprising to note the number of hospitals who are concluding that greater operating room capacity is the sound answer to overall hospital effectiveness — even when they must overcome arguments with state or other reimbursing agencies who mistakenly emphasize individual cost center comparisons to prove their case.

Institutions with high rates of occupancy, in particular, have found that above-normal operating room availability results in fewer OR scheduling problems and more effective bed utilization. For example:

1. Hospitals with ample surgical time rarely, if ever, are forced to postpone elective admissions on days when beds are available, thus avoiding not only empty beds but the frequent loss of the surgeon's time, the disruption of the patient's personal schedule, etc.
2. Previously admitted patients, who have been admitted for diagnosis or for a medical problem that is later found to require surgery, can be accommodated more promptly.
3. Finally, ample operating room time means that more patients can be operated on early in the day, thereby significantly increasing the chances of their being released with one fewer night of hospital stay. (Morning surgery patients are returned to their room by the afternoon and, in many cases, are able to begin the process of returning to normal functions that same day, whereas afternoon surgery patients rarely begin that process until the following day.)

Hospitals with lower occupancy face the "double squeeze" of bed availability and OR availability far less frequently. For them, the cost/benefit ratio of expanding OR capacity would not seem to be as attractive. Nonetheless, some of these hospitals maintain large numbers of operating rooms and a flexible staff in order to accommodate present fluctuations in demand for OR time and future increases in volume. But, without adequate flexibility in staffing the operating room suite, this strategy is exceedingly costly.

APPROACHES TO PROVIDING ADDITIONAL OPERATING ROOM TIME

Hospitals are providing increased operating room time by a variety of methods.

1. Some are extending the hours for elective surgery on weekdays and Saturdays. See Table III-4. Saturday schedules are used primarily for relatively minor procedures, but there is no medical hesitancy about performing major operations on that day. Sunday is restricted to emergency operations at all of the hospitals we visited.
2. A few are carrying out very minor surgery in "lumps and bumps" rooms that are less costly than regular operating rooms to build and operate. Because of the ready availability of regular operating room facilities and personnel in the event of complications, many doctors and patients are finding this a very satisfactory substitute for regular operating rooms.
3. A few have developed or are developing dedicated one-day surgical units to handle most, if not all, of their outpatient and one-day surgical patients, thereby freeing the regular operating rooms for the requirements of inpatients. As the number and type of outpatient operations have increased dramatically, this has made increasing amounts of operating room time available.
4. Some hospitals are building additional regular operating suites or have done so as part of recent renovation projects or expansion programs.
5. Some are providing more effectively available operating time by devoting greater attention to operating room scheduling and management.

SURGICAL SCHEDULING TECHNIQUES

Although the techniques employed for scheduling elective surgery are fundamentally similar, they vary widely in detail — reflecting the fact that none is considered to be completely satisfactory by the surgeons or hospitals involved. Complexities in communications play a large part. In every case, the doctor's office is required to call the hospital to obtain both a

TABLE III–4

OR Availability for Elective Cases

Monday — Friday

Elective Schedule Terminates

Before 5 p.m.	8 Hospitals
To 5 p.m.	1 Hospital
To 5:30 p.m.	2 Hospitals
To 6 p.m.	3 Hospitals
To 7 p.m.	1 Hospital

Saturday

No Saturday surgery	8 Hospitals
Saturday morning only	3 Hospitals
Saturday all day	2 Hospitals
Information not specified	2 Hospitals

Sunday

No elective surgery schedule	15 Hospitals

room reservation and an OR time. At one hospital, this can be fully accomplished in one conversation with one scheduling clerk. However, at several other institutions, mutiple calls and confirmations are required before the physician's office has a confirmed OR time and room reservation.

The system which appears to function most satisfactorily is as follows: Both the admitting and operating room scheduling are performed in a single admitting department office. The admitting department head, a former supervisor in the OR who deals effectively with surgeons, takes an active role in the OR scheduling function. Scheduling clerks receive careful training to assure complete familiarity with the daily routines, physical layout, and special characteristics of the operating room suite. Using two scheduling books simultaneously, the scheduling clerk makes an admitting reservation and schedules a time for surgery. This is the only call required from the physician's office. If changes in the OR schedule become necessary, the scheduling clerk or department head takes the initiative for working it out.

On the day prior to surgery, the admitting department sends a typed surgical schedule to the OR for review. On the day of surgery, last-minute changes (cancellations, emergencies, etc.) are handled by the OR supervisor or head nurse. Physician objections to this system center on its inability to anticipate last-minute changes and thereby prevent inconvenience to the surgeon. The inconvenience factor seems to exist at all hospitals, regardless of their respective systems, and its elimination does not appear to be based on realistic expectations. It is our feeling that many other scheduling systems are overly complex and cumbersome. The greatest number and most severe problems occur where there are complicated systems coupled with high demand and a "passive process" of simply scheduling cases on a first-come, first-serve basis.

OPERATING ROOM MANAGEMENT

Several institutions (including some with the more complex scheduling procedures described above), have taken other steps to refine and manage OR scheduling in order to improve flexibility and maximize productivity. Noteworthy programs include the following:

1. *Physician director* — After several years of widespread frustration with the way the daily surgery schedule was established and managed, the surgeons, nurses, and administrators at one hospital agreed upon a unique and, thus far, successful method of resolving most of the problems. Here an older and widely-respected surgeon has been appointed director of operating room services. A long-time vocal critic of the operating room schedule and of the lack of forceful management in the area, the new director of OR services (now retired as an active surgeon) was quick to acknowledge the value of "co-opting your critics." In his new role, he became responsible to the hospital administration for the management of the OR. He also became involved in decisions to alter the OR schedule (adding cases, moving patients up, etc.) and discussed these and other operational problems with staff surgeons. Perhaps most important, this surgeon had a long and unblemished personal record of promptness for surgical cases and could reprimand other surgeons for being late far more effectively than could any layman. Although he had held his new position for a relatively short time when we visited, it seemed clear that other surgeons were pleased with his results. We noted that he was already working with the hospital's management engineer to develop guidelines for minimizing the time between cases.

2. *Professional manager* — Another hospital concluded that the task of scheduling and managing the nonmedical aspects of operating rooms is one that requires a professional manager rather than the

traditional nursing supervisor or a physician director. The individual selected has an educational background and personality that allows him to manage the OR staff and to interact effectively with physicians. The fact that he is a male is frequently mentioned as a factor that eliminates doctors' traditional tendencies to consider nurses as subordinates.

3. *Time requirement studies* — Over extended time periods, several institutions have carefully monitored the amount of time each surgeon requires to perform specific types of surgery. They have found that by scheduling on the basis of the past practice of specific surgeons, they can prepare operating room schedules that are (a) more realistic and (b) more efficient. Increased efficiency is achieved by avoiding the use of general estimates that include large amounts of precautionary time that, in most cases, is unused.

4. *Odd-even rationing of surgery time* — In one hospital, the surgeons are divided across departmental lines into "red" and "blue" teams. One team may only schedule elective surgery on Monday and Wednesday, while the other is assigned to Tuesday and Thursday. Any surgeons may schedule an elective case on Friday, partially in order to encourage full use of this day. This institution feels that the system equalizes access to surgery time and reduces the chances of a fluctuating surgery schedule throughout the week.

5. *Simultaneous educational meetings* — At a number of institutions, educational conferences for operating room personnel are scheduled to coincide with the educational meetings of the surgical departments. In this way, all educational activity is accomplished without reducing or interrupting the operating schedule.

6. *Limited advance bookings* — In order to prevent surgeons in the more elective fields (orthopedics, ophthalmology, plastic surgery, etc.) from booking all of the prime-time morning surgery months in advance, one hospital places strict daily limits on the number of cases that may be booked in advance by a specific clinical department. However, when unrequested time slots are released seven days before the actual date, these physicians may request remaining time. An important secondary effect of this policy is that the load on specialized nursing units is spread out by reducing or preventing "bunching" in the early days of the week.

7. *Blocked-time scheduling* — Two hospitals function with "blocked time" systems in their operating rooms. In one, access to surgery time is based upon the number of cases performed by each individual surgeon in the prior year. In the other hospital, group practice predominates and scheduling priority is based upon prior group uti-

lization. The latter hospital believes that group scheduling simplifies problems for the hospital, in part because much of the scheduling activity must be carried out by each of the doctor groups with its own personnel. However, the net results are perceived to be an increase in flexibility and a greater likelihood that, with few scheduling units, operating room time will be used more efficiently. An additional benefit of block scheduling by groups rather than by individuals is said to be that the hospital does not become involved in questions regarding the treatment of new physicians since, as a member of an established group, a new surgeon immediately has some access to favorable operating time.

Nonetheless, it is our conclusion that, in spite of the favorable reactions of these hospitals, blocked-time scheduling is significantly less efficient than a free-access system from the perspective of the hospital, and it is less equitable to physicians. It appears to us that the opportunities for less-than-complete utilization of OR time are too great to overcome unless the release date is set sufficiently far in advance so that blocked-time scheduling is not much more than an early reservation priority.

8. *Saturday surgery* — A few hospitals make operating room time available for elective cases on Saturday. Where available, it is normally well utilized. Available time ranges from one room on Saturday morning in some hospitals to one hospital that runs six of its eight operating rooms all day. In that hospital, heavy utilization of the operating rooms on Saturday is accounted for, in part, by the high ratio of surgical procedures to operating rooms even with the extended schedule. It also has proven to be an attractive time for a substantial number of doctors and their patients. And, it has a clearly positive effect on weekend occupancy.

Although two hospitals are considering it, none has begun to perform elective surgery on Sunday. Similarly, no hospital visited has expanded its elective surgery schedule into the evening hours. (However, one hospital began providing one elective room until 7 P.M. as of September 1979.) Most people interviewed felt that surgeons would probably make no more than limited use of these extended periods unless the pressure for OR time was very strong. They seem to feel that a fuller Saturday schedule is the preferable alternative.

DEDICATED FACILITIES FOR MINOR SURGERY

One of the more interesting developments in the management of operating rooms has been the creating of dedicated facilities for the performance of minor surgery for outpatient or one-day surgical patients. As has been previously mentioned, three hospitals have such facilities. They are separate from the major operating suite, relatively more modest, but functionally very satisfactory for the purposes they serve. They are on the same campus as the main hospital, although not necessarily in the same building. Access to the main OR suite is uniformly easy in infrequent cases where back-up services are required.

Physicians and administrators state that the dedicated facilities have the following advantages for both the hospital and the surgeons:

1. Total operating time is expanded at a lower capital cost than is required if the number of major operating rooms is increased.
2. The time available for major operations is increased not only by the removal of the time taken up by the minor operations themselves, but also by the reduction in the clean-up and preparation periods associated with them. One administrator put it this way:

> We used to have a five-week waiting period here for elective surgery ...but [now it is]...one or two days at the most, depending on your time requirement. If you're determined you've got to work at eight o'clock in the morning, then I may not be able to handle that as easily. But even there, we can probably book you in two or three days at the exact time.

   Fewer and longer major surgery cases also reduce the frequency with which patients or surgeons create delays through late arrival.
3. Staffing and operational procedures that are oriented exclusively toward minor surgery are simpler and less expensive than those associated with major surgery. An operating room handling major and minor cases almost inevitably (and necessarily) treats each operation as major. As a consequence, a considerable cost differential exists. This can be used to establish rates for minor surgery that are competitively advantageous. One hospital offers a single, all-inclusive fee based upon type of case. Another offers three categories with charges for the use of the ambulatory surgery room, scaled from a top of $150 down to $50 for a very minor procedure, plus modest additional charges for the recovery room (if it is used) and for supplies.
4. Scheduling of major elective cases is facilitated by removing minor surgery since more operating time is available for that purpose. In addition, more of that time is prime operating time because: minor elective cases are often scheduled weeks or months in advance, when early morning surgical time is still readily available; major surgery generally is scheduled closer to the date on which it is to be performed. If the preferred early morning time has been fully booked

with elective cases, major cases must be done later in the day. Worse, relatively urgent inpatient cases may be delayed for several days before adequate time is available on the surgery schedule.

5. Much of the uncertainty associated with the scheduling of minor surgery is removed. Minor surgery can often be scheduled far in advance, because it is elective in nature and not of particular urgency. By the same token, this makes minor surgery vulnerable to preemption by emergency and even urgent cases, often to the considerable inconvenience of doctor and patient. The risk is substantially reduced, if not eliminated, by the dedicated facility since that facility would be preempted only under very extreme conditions.

Undoubtedly, the number of major operating rooms and their percentage of utilization have a good deal to do with establishing the point at which dedicated one-day surgical facilities should be considered. Such facilities do seem to have a number of advantages and to be at a stage of development where additional improvements should be anticipated.

We looked forward to finding one-day surgery units (or "surgicenters") at off-campus sites. We did not do so, although we did find that several hospitals have established — and subsidized — what amount to be well-developed doctors' offices where very minor surgery (at essentially the "lumps and bumps" level) is performed. These are situated in developing, frequently rural areas, and have been established, in part, for competitive reasons.

UTILIZATION REVIEW

Utilization review efforts are rarely directed toward the surgical operation itself, even though substantial variations exist in the duration of surgical procedures. This situation prevails even when a shortage of operating room time exists. The reasons appear to be:

1. OR time represents a small portion of a patient's hospital stay.
2. It is the most critical point of patient care.
3. Changes forced on the doctor in this area could be very unsettling.
4. The effort could be counterproductive by creating resistance to changes of greater importance for the total length of stay, in which the doctors' cooperation is essential.

As we have previously mentioned, some OR managers and schedulers take variations in surgeon time into account in setting up operating room schedules.

Of at least as great significance, managers and doctors having overall OR management responsibilities do not accept or condone lost time due to the persistent late arrival of specific surgeons or other forms of casual disregard for schedules. However, the extent and success of efforts made to correct the situation seem to vary considerably from hospital to hospital.

PHYSICAL THERAPY SERVICES

No hospital offers anything close to a full range of physical therapy services on weekends. In fact, with one exception, no hospital provides *any* inpatient physical therapy services on either Saturday or Sunday. The reasons given are consistent — cost of additional personnel, insufficient demand due to low occupancy, inability to attract staff to work on weekends, etc. In the one institution where weekend physical therapy services are provided, they are limited to Saturdays. A recent survey of patients at that hospital showed that, over a period of four weeks, 80 percent of the inpatients who routinely required physical therapy treatment, received it on Saturday. However, while the average patient received 1.71 visits on Friday, those same patients received only 1.36 visits on Saturday. On Sunday, no physical therapy services were provided.

We were frequently told by physicians that when these services are not available, the course of patient care slows down. In-house patients, denied a continuation or initiation of therapy over the weekend, not only lose time in the recuperative process but often actually regress. The result is that progress is delayed and length of stay prolonged. For this reason, some orthopedic surgeons indicate a reluctance to perform surgery at the end of the week and, instead, attempt to perform their operations on Monday and Tuesday. The result is to push weekend occupancy lower and occupancy on the most difficult of the weekdays even higher. It also discourages use of the operating rooms near the end of the week. All of these factors are detrimental to maintaining a consistently high level of occupancy.

Significant opportunities seem to exist for improving length of stay and increasing the intensity of care simply by providing physical therapy services on Saturday and Sunday. Although we were surprised that only one institution currently provides this service on Saturday, this program has been such a success that the institution intends to initiate Sunday service in the near future.

PATIENT TRANSPORT AND SCHEDULING

One of the original objectives of our study was to identify ways of improving the physical transport of patients throughout our own hospital.

We looked upon this as one of our special problems, essentially unrelated to the central aim of this study. However, it quickly became clear that transportation of patients within a hospital is an important aspect of a larger problem — that of coordinating inpatient scheduling for ancillary services — as well as a more limited problem in its own right.

In numerous institutions, people described to us the increasing problems involved in timing all the services an individual patient uses in a given day (physical therapy, radiology, respiratory therapy, EKG, etc.). It was underscored that efficient scheduling and coordination of tests and services is imperative in order to prevent conflicts that reduce the operating efficiency of the individual departments and, where delays or postponements occur, slow the course of patient care. Clearly, as average length of stay is reduced by other means, scheduling problems for ancillary services are aggravated as the attending physician and the hospital try to compress more activity into the individual patient's day. This is a problem which just now appears to be gaining attention in most of the hospitals we visited.

We observed two attempts (one ambitious and one simple) to coordinate the schedules of various departments to accommodate the total needs of the individual patient. One institution is attempting to develop a central scheduling office that would coordinate the tests and treatments ordered for a given patient in a way that would eliminate conflicts and minimize the degree to which other patient activities (meals, visiting hours, sleep) were interrupted. All ancillary departments finalize their work schedules through this office, which also provides the necessary transport personnel.

The other hospital is attempting to achieve essentially the same result at the level of the individual nursing unit. A large magnetic board, with patient names on the vertical axis and time intervals along the horizontal axis, is placed directly across from each nursing station. As individual activities are scheduled for specific patients, the unit clerk blocks off the appropriate time slot for that patient with a coded magnet. This avoids conflicts and permits any staff member to see where a patient should be at any given time. However, this system has two problems. First, it depends on the unit clerk's diligence and accuracy in posting appointments and changes. Second, it compromises confidentiality by posting all the patients' names in a prominent place.

It is our impression that much can be gained by successful efforts in coordinating the patient-related activities in all ancillary departments, both in terms of operating efficiency and patient convenience. But the solution, while straightforward, is not simple, because of the detail and extensive communications involved. The internal transport of patients, considered in its more limited sense, remains a chronic, unresolved, frequently studied problem with an approximately even split between centralized transport departments and systems where individual departments have their own transport personnel. About the same number of advantages and disadvantages are cited on both sides.

Centralized transport systems generally are said to lack the ability to respond appropriately to unusual situations in a particular department and to lack accountability to ancillary department heads for bringing patients for treatment on a timely basis. *Decentralized* transport systems are characterized as more expensive, less efficient, and less able to assure that patients move through treatments and tests involving multiple departments as quickly and with as little inconvenience as possible.

The only development encountered of particular note uses volunteers much more successfully than the norm, particularly with respect to the admitting function. Here, according to the hospital Chief Executive Officer (CEO):

> [We have] probably fifteen volunteers [a day, including] Saturday. They handle the whole admitting process. They escort the patients upstairs; they introduce the patient to the nurse on the floor; and they stay with that patient until they turn him over to a nurse. The volunteers run their own training program for new recruits every month.

THE AVAILABILITY OF CONSULTANTS*

Physicians in several hospitals with short lengths of stay attribute it, in part, to their ability to obtain consultations quickly from specialists on the medical staff. This occurs because (1) all of the appropriate specialties are represented on the medical staff, (2) they are present in sufficient numbers to encourage competition, and (3) there are not too many to preclude development of personal relationships among medical staff members. The physicians believe that these might not be essential elements of satisfactory consulting arrangements, but such conditions have greatly facilitated the development of their own consultations and, most likely, would for other doctors.

From our perspective, consultants fall into two categories: first, hospital-based physicians providing specific services of a diagnostic or therapeutic nature (e.g., pathologists, radiologists, anesthesiologists, physiatrists, and specialists in pulmonary medicine) and second, private practitioners en-

---

* While this discussion does not relate to hospital-based consultants, the topic has been included here because of its similarity to other topics discussed in this section.

gaged primarily or exclusively in a particular subspecialty (e.g., nephrologists, cardiologists, and neurologists). The availability of consultants of the first type is discussed in some detail in the sections dealing with the specific hospital departments (in particular, the laboratory and the radiology departments). The following comments concern the second group of consultants.

Because of the increasing complexity of medicine, today's physicians find themselves dependent upon a variety of specialists whose skills may not have even existed ten or fifteen years ago. The ready availability of these skills has thus become an increasingly important factor in the process of patient care.

Hospitals and physicians appear to be uniform in their desire to have a well-balanced medical staff that includes as many specialties as possible. There is a clear concensus that this is much better than a situation in which outside specialists frequently must be consulted. In part, this is because staff membership brings about greater physical accessibility. But more important are the greater degree of commitment and loyalty that is anticipated and the willingness of the consultant to extend himself on behalf of the doctor and the institution.

On the question of group versus individual practice, opinions are more diverse. In general, there seems to be a feeling that multiple-member, single-specialty groups provide easier access to a greater number of potential specialists and, frequently, expanded hours of coverage. But it is felt that, by reducing competition, a situation is created where some physicians are less inclined to be inconvenienced for a consultation than are a number of solo practitioners or small partnerships. However, the variation in feeling with respect to specific groups and doctors was more important than any conclusion regarding organizational format.

Although findings concerning doctors' office buildings are discussed in a later chapter, it is worth noting at this point that physicians and administrators at three hospitals with on-campus office buildings indicate that the proximity to the hospital and the close working relationship of doctors in those buildings make it easier not only for consultants to see a patient quickly but also for attending physicians to catch the consultant in the corridor, his office, or nearby to obtain advice and assistance. The ready availability of consultants located in on-campus office buildings is also said to have been helpful to doctors whose own offices are sprinkled throughout several towns.

IV

Facilitating the
Efficient Use of the
Hospital by Attending Physicians

It is logical that doctors, individually and collectively, should have the greatest impact on a hospital's rate of occupancy and length of stay. They decide who should be admitted, how the patient will be treated, and when the patient should be discharged. It is often said that the most expensive piece of equipment in a modern hospital is a doctor's pen. With it he can order the admission or the discharge of a patient as well as an infinite variety of tests, examinations, treatments, and procedures. In short, with his pen the doctor can quickly and easily commit massive resources and spend thousands of dollars on behalf of a patient.

While expensive hospital hardware and the ways in which it is used gather most of the headlines and consume the greatest interest of Health Systems Agencies and other regulatory bodies, the physician's decision to admit a patient and the timing of his subsequent decision to discharge that patient have a far greater impact on the rate of hospital use and health care costs than all of the so-called "exotic" tests combined.

All doctors acknowledge that custom, training, science, and environment all play a part in these determinations, that their actions vary with circumstances, and that, by and large, the lengths of stay for comparable patients have declined considerably over the past ten years. They cite a variety of reasons for this reduction. Some, such as better diagnostic equipment, more powerful medicines, new surgical techniques, and the like, represent improvements in the tools available to doctors. Other reasons relate to the manner in which hospital-based doctors and employees provide medical, physical, and administrative support to doctors' efforts. Still other reasons, such as a greater appreciation of the value of early ambulation (instead of inactive bed care), changes in cultural attitudes, bed-shortage pressures, regulatory requirements, utilization reviews, and similar factors, are more judgmental and intangible in nature. As Griffith, Hancock and Munson state in their introduction to *Cost Control in Hospitals:*

> We believe that the doctor decides who should be admitted based upon the situation he faces. The availability of alternatives to admission, the occupancy level, the delays and inconvenience surrounding admission and service, the payment mechanism, and the attitudes of his peers influence that decision as well as the patient's needs and attitudes. Systems which raise hospital occupancy, guarantee admission dates, and encourage preadmission testing affect the length of stay directly and influence the admission decision at least indirectly. We believe that these systems facilitate still other actions, such as more effective utilization review and more appropriate response to acute hospital substitutes like home care and ambulatory surgery.*

This chapter will focus mainly on length of stay and will deal, in more general terms, with the efficiency and effectiveness with which doctors make use of hospital services and facilities. Headings include:

- Lengths of Stay in the Individual Hospital
- Variations in Lengths of Stay among Hospitals
- Length of Stay in Obstetrical Services
- Some General Comments on Physician Efficiency
- Medical Office Buildings

It will be recognized that, while a number of comments are relevant to mandated mechanisms such as utilization review, they are equally relevant when legal requirements do not exist.

LENGTH OF STAY IN THE INDIVIDUAL HOSPITAL

The importance of the doctor's role in hospital utilization and length of stay has been increasingly recognized in what many doctors would say is both a positive and a negative manner. Doctors have taken the initiative

---

* Griffith, John R.; Hancock, Walton M.; and Munson, Fred C. *Cost Control in Hospitals.* (Ann Arbor, Mich.: Health Administration Press, 1976), p. 5.

in examining and improving their own performance and in working with hospital administrators and trustees to provide services and equipment that help them to do so. Also, doctors are subjected to a variety of controls over patient care — some directed at the average lengths of stay and costs of patients and diagnoses, and others at the admission and treatment of individual patients. Consequently, surveillance mechanisms — medical audits and utilization reviews and PSROs — have been developed, and reimbursement agencies have established methodologies that question the medical judgments of individual doctors by denying payment to the hospital, doctor, or patient for what they consider to be unjustifiable charges. Much of this methodology is backed up by increasingly comprehensive statistical data that highlight differences in physician treatment patterns, length of stay practices, and costs for individual diagnoses, doctors, and patients.

For the most part, the hospitals included in this survey have been able to comply with these requirements without undue difficulty since, by virtue of their selection, their lengths of stay are at the lower end of the scale on the average, if not for all patients, doctors, and diagnoses. Many hospitals and doctors consider the regulations and controls to be essentially ineffective and unnecessary red tape and comply only because they are compelled to do so. They feel they have achieved or would have achieved a short length of stay as a direct consequence of the way that they practice medicine rather than as a result of organized programs or external pressures. For them, such programs constitute what they feel is an unnecessary formalization and they often resent the fact that improvements are attributed to programs that they find distasteful. However, others have achieved substantial results by using the mechanisms — especially utilization review and medical audit — very constructively.

As a generalization, it is fair to state that, where utilization review programs have been well designed, managed, and accepted by physicians, they have had a widespread impact on physicians' perceptions of length of stay and admission requirements. Where utilization programs have not been accepted by physicians, they have had little or no impact. In fact, what impact they may have had could well be negative as physicians react to what they perceive to be regimentation and unnecessary documentation. A few hospitals base their utilization review programs on the rather lengthy norms provided in the Professional Activity Study (PAS) books or selected by PSROs. In such instances, the utilization review is generally credited with achieving only minimal results by:

a. providing physicians with an external focus of blame when they must tell reluctant patients to leave the hospital or face termination of benefits;

  b. leading the few consistently "long-stay physicians" to bring their
     cases in line with the norms to avoid the harassment of disputes,
     extra documentation, etc.; and
  c. reminding the other physicians of potentially excessive stays in very
     occasional situations.

These hospitals have strong doubts about the net merits of the effort.

At the other end of the scale are hospitals that more aggressively use the
approach to achieve substantially greater results. We will describe the elements of these approaches, ignoring for this purpose the many hospitals
that fall in between. The high-achievement systems have the following
characteristics:

  1. They do not use PAS and other relatively low-level standards but
     instead use tighter standards that they or others have developed.
     These standards are based on or reflect historical data, but they usu-
     ally involve elements of selectivity (i.e., weighing the better physi-
     cians performance more heavily) and even of conscious stretching.
     Hospitals using these norms work on the assumption that sound, in-
     ternally developed criteria, when effectively presented, form the
     basis for a highly persuasive argument in changing the practice pat-
     terns of departments and individual physicians. As the medical
     director in one institution commented, "They have to buy it. You
     can show them where they can do better. What else can they do?
     They can't say, 'No, I don't want to do better.'"
  2. They do not restrict utilization review efforts to Medicare, Medi-
     caid, and other cases where it is required but extend it to the entire
     range of patients handled by the hospital as recommended by the
     Joint Commission on the Accreditation of Hospitals (JCAH).
  3. They do not, except where required, apply utilization review to all
     patients. Instead, they use statistical data at their disposal and other
     techniques to identify *specific* problem areas, including patient
     diagnoses and physicians, and apply most of their efforts to improv-
     ing performance there. The basic objective is, as one medical direc-
     tor stated, "to cure the cause of the problem, not just to check spe-
     cific abuses." Under this approach, attention is focused not only on
     individual patients passing through the hospital system but on the
     hospital itself and problems affecting patient stays (e.g., turnaround
     time for laboratory tests).
  4. A substantial portion of their effort is spent on concurrent reviews of
     patients and problems that stimulate the greatest interest. As a con-
     sequence, they check problems as they are developing and deter-

mine the effectiveness of current attempts to implement solutions. In addition, by combining concurrency and selectivity, the interest of the Utilization Review Committee is constantly made evident in a large number of areas.

5. They arrange for a close integration of those concerned with utilization review and medical audit, emphasizing areas of mutual interest and the free flow of useful information between the groups. One instance of this integration resulted in incorporating both the standards and actual results of medical audits into the utilization reviews of specific diagnoses. This has had the effect of integrating considerations of time and quality of care by directing attention to the consequences of excessively short stays, on the one hand, and the costs of excessively long stays on the other. In more than one instance, it also has led to an analysis by a clinical department, with or without the assistance of medical audit, of alternative approaches to particular diagnoses. The result has been the development of "preferred" care plans and standards that influence future behavior of physicians as well as serve as the basis for reviewing future costs and charts.

6. Finally, these programs enlist the interest and participation of the medical staff officers, department directors and, through them, individual doctors at their departmental meetings. It is evident that strong and sustained backing by the leaders of the medical staff is important, not only in the policies they enunciate but in more practical matters such as the selection of doctors for the Utilization Review and Medical Audit Committees. In addition, well-respected doctors who support "the cause" in their formal and informal discussions and by their personal examples are invaluable.

Such supporters are, however, outside the operative chain of command which goes from the utilization review department or its physician advisors to (1) the individual doctor in specific cases or (2) to the medical staff president or the department director in more general situations, as opportunities are tackled for constructive improvement in an entire department's average performance with respect to all or selected diagnoses or the performance of individual doctors.

Hospitals making the more noteworthy achievements attack these opportunities firmly, but with due consideration for the feelings of those affected. They recognize that doctors — not laymen — change doctors. Many do it on a departmental director-to-physician basis, but others discuss length-of-stay problems quite openly at departmental meetings, even when the names of the offending physicians can be guessed or identified. At least one institution encourages broad understanding of the objectives and results of the utilization review program by including a member of the board of trustees on the Utilization Review Committee and by sending a monthly report to the board on the Utilization Review Program and the Quality Assurance Program.

7. Hospitals making the most of these opportunities have utilization review and medical audit personnel who believe strongly in what they are doing. They are people who are recognized for their impartiality and their ability to minimize the difficult personal aspects of their work. They have a wide variety of personal traits. They usually can put whatever knowledge they have to good use, as is evidenced most clearly by one hospital where the very experienced utilization review nurses note inconsistencies between intensity of treatment and discharge plans and follow up on them.

The two most successful utilization review programs are headed by physicians who not only take their positions seriously and currently are or have been competent and respected practitioners but are also leaders and opinion-molders among the medical staff.

Because of the sensitive nature of the position (particularly in a hospital where the program is an aggressive one), it is generally agreed that the utilization review chairman should not be dependent on referrals from other physicians. In one instance, the individual responsible for the utilization review program and its success is the medical director of the hospital. In large part, the widespread support of physicians for the utilization review program at this hospital can be traced to this independence and to the fact that the medical director is viewed by his peers as being truly supportive of both physician and patient. In addition, this medical director has successfully designed the program so that the individual physician is only minimally exposed to one of his least favorite chores — paperwork.

8. Finally, it is clear that hospitals with aggressive programs make extensive use of computer facilities to provide information as to what is occurring, to identify problems, and to let "figures speak" in suggesting to doctors where their attention should be focused and the nature and size of the expected results. Two hospitals have developed extensive and imaginative computer systems to provide physicians, utilization review personnel, and other appropriate individuals with a broad range of information on short notice. This information includes historical analysis of length of stay by diagnosis and physician, cost per case and per diagnosis by physician, utilization of ancillary services by physician by diagnosis, and outcome information. The information is compiled and routinely given

to the physicians on the Utilization Review and Medical Audit Committees in a format that is useful to them. As the lay director of medical education at one institution said:

> If you give smart people information, they'll act on it. You have to make sure that you, the institution, provide the physicians with all the backup that's necessary to get that information, because physicians won't do it. They won't collect it. They're certainly not going to key-punch it into a computer. They'll never read the reports that come out of a computer, but they are interested in the information. So what we've tried to create here is a system by which we gather the data and put it into our computers and get it out of these computers by physician, by floor, by age, by diagnosis, by whatever means we want. . . . Then we have created between the physicians and the computer. . . a system by which we convert that basic data into information. Part of the philosophy is that you do not waste physicians' time. They feel they're getting something out of it when they sit down to review the information.

Most of the institutions are PSRO-delegated. However, three hospitals with aggressive internal programs have chosen not to be delegated. They believe (1) that by assuming all of the PSRO-required work, the capacity of utilization review personnel to perform more sophisticated, focused reviews is greatly diminished and (2) that the confusion resulting from using both the PSRO standards and their own tighter standards simultaneously is avoided. These institutions provide the PSRO employees with office space and permit them to do their reviews of patients admitted under Title XVIII and Title XIX. Because these institutions have lengths of stay substantially below the norms, they do not need to pay much attention to the PSRO employees. Instead, they maintain their own utilization review staffs who continue to review the patients of those physicians who may need encouragement to reduce the length of stay for identified diagnoses. Hospitals that have accepted delegation appear to have strong reservations about it except as a means of keeping more of the hospital's activities under medical staff control.

At two institutions with long-standing utilization review programs, we were told that the recent PSRO delegation had quickly resulted in a diminution of physicians' interest and participation in utilization review activities. In another institution where physicians have never been enthusiastic about utilization review, the institutional length of stay began to climb (after years of dropping), concurrently with PSRO delegation. If the indicated correlations are correct and continue to exist, their implications for the PSRO program are certainly not positive.

One hospital's chief of staff, perhaps expressing hope as much as reality, said, "Most of us feel that PSRO will. . . collapse of its own weight, because of the bureaucracy involved. It just does not fit into the good, economical practice of medicine." The chairman of the Utilization Review Committee at another hospital suggested that an effective compromise might be for the neighboring hospitals to become delegated PSROs for each other.

VARIATIONS IN LENGTHS OF STAY AMONG HOSPITALS

In spite of the substantial decline in length of stay over the past ten years for virtually all hospitals and doctors and in spite of the kinds of efforts previously considered in our discussion of utilization reviews, one important fact remains:

There are often substantial differences among hospitals in the length of stay for comparable diagnoses that cannot be explained by differences in patient characteristics. These differences exist among hospitals in different cities, counties, and states and, to a striking degree, among broad, regional areas of the country.

SOME COMPARATIVE DATA

This point is vividly illustrated by Table IV-1 (page 83), which shows the length of stay (LOS) for twelve frequent diagnoses at The Valley Hospital and the fourteen hospitals visited. What is apparent from the chart is:

1. that substantial variations exist between the high and the low hospitals in every instance,
2. that even the variation between the high and the median hospitals typically ranges from 20 to 40 percent, and
3. that achievements at one hospital for one diagnosis often says little about achievements for other diagnoses.

What cannot be seen from the table because of the manner in which the hospital coding has been disguised is that, in 75 percent of the cases, the LOS of the four hospitals we visited in the western part of the United States were below the median; that, in 60 percent of the cases, their LOS were among the lowest 5; and that, in 40 percent of the cases, they were among the lowest three. While we had seen such information in the aggregate in the AHA's *Hospitals*,* we found it more striking to encounter it

---

* *Hospitals*, Journal of the American Hospital Association, Vol. 55, No. 8 (April 16, 1979), p. 70.

TABLE IV-1

COMPARATIVE LENGTH OF STAY (1978): TWELVE REPRESENTATIVE DIAGNOSES

Myocardial Infarction		Congestive Heart Failure		Delivery		Spontaneous Abortion		Sterilization		Uterine Fibroma	
18.7	H	14.3	F	4.4	M	2.0	C	2.9	K	8.5	A
17.1	A	14	D	4.2	H	2.0	F	2.9	J	8.4	H
17.1	B	13.9	A	4.0	F	2.0	I	2.4	B	8.1	B
17	D	12.7	K	4	O	2	D	2.4	E	8	D
16.4	K	12.1	M	3.9	E	1.8	G	2.3	I	7.8	C
15.9	M	12.1	N	3.8	N	1.6	M	1.8	G	7.4	M
15.8	F	12.0	H	3.7	A	1.6	O	1.6	M	7	O
15.4	C	11	B	3.5	C	1.5	E	1.4	O	6.9	E
13.9	N	10.6	C	3.4	K	1.5	K	1	D	6.5	J
13.1	G	10	O	3.0	J	1.2	A	1.0	N	6.3	L
12.4	E	9.6	E	3	D	1.2	L			6.1	F
12.2	L	9.5	I	2.6	G	1.1	N			5.7	I
12	O	9.2	G	2.6	I	1.1	J			5.4	G
11.8	J	8.1	L	1.8	L	1.0	B			5.0	N
10.8	I	7.6	J			1.0	H			4.2	K
Range* 73%		88%		144%		100%		190%		102%	

Inguinal Hernia		Choleli- thiasis		Lumbo Sacral Spr. & Strain		Displ. Int. Disc		Cataract		Hypertrophy Tonsils	
5.0	B	11.2	M	9.9	M	14.0	K	6.0	B	2.2	C
5.0	M	10.8	A	9.8	N	13.6	F	5.0	I	2.2	A
5	D	10.3	B	9.0	H	13.4	M	4.9	M	2.0	F
4.8	C	10	D	8.8	G	13	D	4.7	K	2	D
4.8	G	9.9	K	8.6	F	13	O	3.9	F	1.9	E
4.5	A	9.6	F	7.0	B	12.4	B	3.7	C	1.8	G
4.3	L	9.6	L	7	D	12	A	3.7	N	1.8	J
4.0	F	9.5	E	7	O	11.6	C	3.2	A	1.8	O
4.0	H	9.2	C	6.5	J	11.6	L	3	D	1.7	I
4	O	9	O	6.2	C	11	H	3	O	1.5	M
3.8	I	8.8	G	6.0	K	10.6	N	2.9	G	1.4	K
3.5	E	8.5	N	6.0	L	10.3	G	2.8	E	1.3	B
3.5	J	8.0	H	5.9	A	9.2	I	2.8	L	1.3	L
3.5	N	7.9	I	5.8	I	8.1	E	2.7	J	1.1	H
3.5	K	6.3	J			7.4	J	1.0	H	1.0	N
Range* 43%		78%		71%		89%		500%		120%	

Note: Letter code following each numerical value represents a hospital.

* Percentage difference between the highest and the lowest length of stay

in actual practice in specific institutions much like our own. The similarity of western LOS data in the face of the widely diverse conditions in which the four western hospitals we visited operate, the lower overall averages for the western region presented in *Hospitals*, and the existence of substantially lower PAS length-of-stay standards for western states indicate that western LOS cannot be accounted for by easy factors such as age and climate. The fact is that there *is* a substantial difference between the West and the rest of the country and that evidence of it seems to indicate a significant opportunity for other hospitals throughout the nation. Doctors with whom we talked, several of whom had moved to the West after completing their training or, in a few cases, from an established career in other sections of the country, confirmed that shorter LOS does, in fact, exist in the West. They stated that the basic treatment of a given diagnosis was comparable, that the diagnostic or preoperative period was essentially similar, and that the difference could be found primarily in the recovery period.

"They just go home sooner" was the frequent explanation, but, at times, it was expressed in more vivid terms:

> We are quite upset with the differences around the United States. When I was utilization chairman, being basically a rabble rouser, I tried to incite revolutionary feelings among my colleagues because we were quite distressed to see the difference in allotments of time back East. And when you realize that half of the men on the staff trained on the other side of the Mississippi River, it's a source of annoyance to us that the patients of the colleagues who were misled and headed east, instead of heading west, get twice or almost twice in some instances, the length of stay that ours get.

The situation in Tucson, where 60 percent of the mothers and babies born in uncomplicated births go home the day after birth, is the most dramatic difference noted. But, in this instance as in others, we were advised that both undesirable aftereffects of early discharge and required readmissions are minimal. The overwhelming proportion of patients simply spend less time in the hospital with no ill effects.

Differences in the length of stay of acute myocardial infarction (MI) patients are in many ways equally dramatic. Although nationwide figures indicate an average LOS of 15–17 days for acute MIs, the hospitals studied range from 10.8 to 18.7 days. *All* of the western hospitals are well below the median. Our study's findings are supported in a comparison of recently completed length-of-stay studies for the western United States, California only, and the mid-Atlantic region. While more than 42,000 acute MI patients in the mid-Atlantic region stayed an average of 17.0

days* in 1977–1978, 21,600 western-states patients stayed 13.8 days in 1976** and some 8,300 California patients stayed 10.9 days in 1977.***

THE OPPORTUNITY FOR IMPROVEMENT

How the substantially lower western LOS came about is not as important as the fact that it exists. There certainly have been many factors. Undoubtedly, bed shortages in the past played a part. Undoubtedly, the generally fluid and innovative cultures of certain parts of the West have been important in creating new ideas with respect to medical care and gaining community acceptance of them. And, undoubtedly, the Kaiser-Permanente Plan and the rapid and continuing growth of HMOs and similar organizations have introduced important elements of competition and of economic self-interest on the part of doctors. The significant fact, however, is that low lengths of stay are a part of the current expectations of the medical and patient communities and that these lengths of stay are continuing to drop even in the face of substantial oversupply of hospital beds in most hospitals and most communities.

It would clearly seem that hospitals and their medical staffs throughout the country would perform a substantial service to their hospitals and communities by adopting — or at least consciously moving significantly toward — the LOS practices of western hospitals. This undoubtedly would involve a general lowering of LOS for most doctors and a concerted effort to change the relatively few doctors in almost every hospital whose patients consistently exceed the hospital average to a substantial extent.

Part of the process of making a significant change of this nature involves the creation of a new set of expectations on the part of those affected — in this case, the medical, hospital, and patient communities. Some changes in expectations will undoubtedly have to take place before actual improvement occurs but, given a gradual rate of change, others undoubtedly will take place as a result of the improvements.

---

* Hospital Utilization Project, *HUP Length of Stay: 1977–1978, Mid-Atlantic Region* (Pittsburg, Penn.: 1979), p. 52.

** Commission on Professional and Hospital Activities, *Length of Stay in PAS Hospitals by Diagnosis, Western Region, 1976* (Ann Arbor, Mich.: 1977), p. 90.

*** McDonnell Douglas Corporation, *California Length of Stay, 1977* (Hazelwood, Missouri: 1978), p. 5–192.

LACK OF KNOWLEDGE OF COMPARATIVE LENGTH-OF-STAY DATA

The above discussion argues, first, for a greater awareness of the length-of-stay records of other hospitals and, second, for the development of goals and programs for bringing about changes in individual hospitals. We would like to comment briefly on the first item on the basis of our survey.

We were surprised by the lack of knowledge about lengths of stay that we encountered in virtually every hospital including our own. There is always an extensive amount of information available about one's own hospital or local group of hospitals. There is also a great deal of information about some larger geographical area, most often an HSA area or state, but it tends to obscure outstanding performance by the use of averages and the combination of data into major categories that are not specific enough to be very useful. And, by taking a local or parochial view, the hospital does not avail itself of information about what is going on in other more distant parts of the country.

In short, most hospitals have access to information about the overall LOS data of other hospitals that, although often confusing and even computed on different bases, is generally indicative of overall hospital performance. The weakness of this data, for the purposes we are discussing, lies in its generality. More specific data is needed to identify problems and opportunities — and expectations — in terms that affect individual doctors and their patients.

The extent to which we found eastern and midwestern hospitals unaware of western LOS data and both the surprise and the generally positive actions that this data produced are important indicators of its potential value. Of further interest is the lack of knowledge of the wide disparity of performance in and among high-quality nonwestern hospitals. Both factors lend support to the concept that information about remarkable LOS performance — whether gained through statistical analyses or interhospital visits by members of the medical staff — is critical in developing new sets of expectations, based upon the demonstrated accomplishments of leading doctors and institutions. It likewise strongly supports the idea that information about shorter LOS performance should *not*, as it presently is, be restricted to a few, mostly utilization review doctors, but be made more widely available and the subject of widespread discussion. Noteworthy is the fact that, in several hospitals where substantial progress has been made in dealing with LOS problems, useful information is available and received serious consideration at departmental meetings. Without this type of constant infusion of information regarding developments in this area and an organized way of incorporating them into a hospital's expectations and standards, even the better hospitals run a great risk of becoming dated and parochial.

TEACHING INSTITUTIONS AND LENGTH OF STAY

Because we intended to visit hospitals whose key characteristics were similar to our own, we minimized the number of teaching hospitals selected. One of these exceptions was a midwestern teaching hospital whose LOS achievements were noteworthy in relation to both teaching and nonteaching hospitals in its areas. At that institution, a long-standing attitude, fostered and encouraged by the hospital, places a high value on efficient and rapid inpatient care. This is instilled into the residents and has resulted in a uniform belief among people at this hospital that their teaching program results in a lower length of stay. This is obviously contradictory to conventional wisdom about teaching programs resulting in longer LOS. However, this conventional wisdom is categorically rejected by the physicians and the administrators of this institution. A leading surgeon at this hospital put it this way:

> I don't think that because you're training interns, residents, etc., you keep the patient around longer at all. In fact, I think that if you're going to train them well, you've got to train them a little bit in economy. . . . Surgeons around here pride themselves on selectivity in arriving at a diagnosis — what one of the speakers at [a recent] meeting called "elegance of diagnosis": the fewest number of studies that will accurately pinpoint the diagnosis or get you to the point where you can act on the patient's behalf. . . . So I don't think the presence of a house staff should increase length of stay and my personal feeling is that it may help shorten it. . . . They [the residents] are the ones who advertise. . . "Hey, Dr. W———'s letting his gall bladders go home on the third day instead of the sixth. . . or fifth day and they seem to be doing all right." What the hell! I'm as good as [Dr.] W———. . . . I can let mine go too and I think it can help.

CONCLUSION REGARDING LENGTH OF STAY

It would be quite incorrect to conclude that serious interest in and efforts toward reducing length of stay are concentrated in western hospitals, for we encountered them throughout the country. What impressed us so greatly was the general level of current achievement and the casualness with which it is accepted and the firm expectation that further reductions will be achieved in the future — perhaps even in some of the diagnoses that Table IV-1 indicates as being most productive.

It is our belief that the biggest single opportunity for most hospitals to reduce their LOS lies in implementing the patient-management practices employed in western hospitals. Clearly, attitude and expectations, supported by information, are an important part of a move in that direction.

LENGTH OF STAY IN OBSTETRICAL SERVICES

Two aspects of obstetrical services stand out vividly:

1. the wide differences in length of stay, varying between a low of 1.8 days for an uncomplicated birth in one western hospital to 4.4 days at a hospital in the East, and
2. the varying fortunes of different hospitals, falling along a spectrum extending from large and expanding volumes to complete discontinuance.

REASONS FOR VARIATIONS

The present variations in length of stay appear to result from a variety of attitudes held by physicians and patients, from economic pressures, and to a lesser extent, from hospital practices. Obviously, these variations largely depend on the judgment of the doctor as to the ability of the mother and baby to leave the hospital and utilize external follow-up measures. It is our understanding that doctors with short-stay obstetrical patients are confident (1) that most mothers can return home after one or two days and (2) that those who should remain for a longer period can readily be identified. These doctors feel that by erring on the conservative side, readmissions and other problems can be held to levels that are equal to or lower than those found in longer-stay hospitals. Furthermore, they feel that there are advantages in removing mother and child from a potentially infectious environment. They recognize that there are advantages in having the baby under surveillance during the first few days but feel that the principal potential problem — jaundice caused by bilirubin imbalance — can be detected from a blood sample taken during a doctor's office visit on the third day or, in some cases, even with questions asked by a nurse or doctor in a telephone call. These doctors also rely to some extent on the education of the mother before birth and in the hospital by means of "mothering" classes.

Those who believe in a longer LOS basically prefer to minimize medical risks through providing hospital care during a longer period under conditions that also are more convenient for the doctors involved. Obstetricians whose patients have longer lengths of stay frequently acknowledge that they consider the last day or two of the stay to be essentially rest for the mother, providing a time for physical recovery and psychological pleasure before facing the rigors of family life, especially when the baby is not the firstborn.

Psychological attitudes are also important in determining OB lengths of stay. Doctors state that many patients who desire to return home quickly do so simply because they prefer a home setting to the hospital. They may also prefer a birthing room (found in seven of the hospitals visited) to the more clinical atmosphere of a delivery room, and they may prefer to start or continue the bonding of baby and family in a natural environment as soon as possible. Such attitudes are said to be widespread and growing.

Economic factors are also of substantial importance, particularly for young parents, who usually lack the financial resources necessary to stay beyond the period provided by insurance contracts.* It is not surprising that there is a direct correlation between insurance coverage and length of stay and that the strength of the influence of HMOs and similar sophisticated group purchasers is also reflected in the LOS practices of different areas. Each acts to condition parents, doctors, and hospitals.

Availability of Mothering Classes

Other aspects of hospital practice affecting occupancy and LOS also deserve mention. The first involves the establishment of a safety factor for late admittances and the handling of peak loads in mixed OB/GYN units (see page 17 for a discussion of these matters). The second involves the availability of "mothering" classes, which are presented at many of the hospitals. These classes are considered to be an important part of the mother's stay and of her preparation in taking care of the baby at home.

Two hospitals conduct mothering classes on the maternity unit at least once a day. One supplements its classes with a series of video-tape cassettes, which individuals may watch at their own convenience right on the postpartum unit, and provides opportunities to obtain answers from the nurses to questions that the tapes raise. In these institutions, all new mothers promptly receive appropriate training and can be discharged as soon as their medical condition permits. At least one of these hospitals also has its nurses make one or more follow-up telephone calls to the mother at

---

* In some areas, limited capitation payments by insurance companies (particularly Blue Cross) for obstetrical stays place the financial burden directly on any patient who stays more than two days without medically justifiable reasons. Obviously, this is a great incentive for short lengths of stay.

home during the first few days in order to offer advice or answer questions.*

Individuals at other hospitals indicate that the lack of mothering classes or their relatively infrequent presentation (i.e., only three days per week and never on weekends) often causes a new mother and her physician to delay discharge by at least a day, solely for this purpose. When one considers the cost per day of hospital care for both mother and baby, this is clearly an expensive practice.

Length of Stay and the Closing of Obstetrical Departments

Another matter deserves discussion here. While the fate of the obstetrical units of numerous individual hospitals is uncertain, it is evident that direct regulations and unfavorable economic returns are going to force a large number of low-volume obstetrical departments out of existence. If this occurs, a strong possibility exists that a disproportionate share of doctors and births will go to the more popular and successful hospitals where the volume of births may already be creating a high rate of occupancy. The trend toward a greater proportion of Caesarean sections may increase bed requirements further. Thus, the extent to which other doctors and patients can be accommodated may directly relate to the extent this is permitted by the average length of stay.

Some General Comments on Physician Efficiency

Comments in the preceding three sections touched only lightly on an important aspect of one topic — the substantial variations that apparently exist in the ability of, or the effort expanded by, individual doctors to utilize the hospital and its services efficiently. This is not a phenomenon that we observed firsthand. Rather, it was brought to our attention in numerous interviews with chiefs of staff, attending physicians, and ancillary-department doctors, directors of nursing, and others. Their comments run along the following lines:

The ability of and efforts made by individual doctors to use the scope of services offered by the hospital in an efficient manner differ for a wide variety of reasons. Medical skills and competence are obviously involved in the ability to diagnose patient problems quickly and ac-

---

* Historically, these nurses also made a visit to the patient's home. However, problems with liability insurance coverage caused the termination of such a program.

curately, with a minimum number of tests. And so is the ability to lay out a course of treatment that will accomplish a great deal in a short space of time. Beyond that, there are numerous factors that affect the ease and frequency with which the doctor uses the hospital — nature of practice, location of office, number of hospital affiliations, etc. But even when conditions are equal, effectiveness varies greatly for the following reasons:

1. Some doctors are better organized than others, as is reflected in their working habits. One noticeable difference in their use of the hospital is the extent to which they have thought out the patient's problems in advance and the diagnostic procedures they intend to follow, given the alternative findings of the various tests. In fact, a small number of doctors, when the diagnostic procedures are time-consuming or require special facilities or doctors, schedule the most probable sequence of tests in advance of or shortly after admission, taking care that the sequence does not result in delays because of chemical inconsistencies.

2. Some doctors work exceedingly well with the principal ancillary departments. They draw on the substantial skills of these departments, consulting with them in advance to develop a diagnostic program that will minimize the number of tests ordered and conflicts in test sequences. Pathologists, in particular, point out this opportunity although radiologists in one hospital are presently reexamining their testing strategy to determine when it is best to move directly to a final test, e.g., a brain or body scan, and eliminate most of the intermediate procedures. They request expedited tests when they both need and will use them promptly. Alternatively, they plan their hospital rounds with the availability of test information in mind.

3. Some doctors obtain consultations with a minimum of patient delay.

4. Some doctors take the time and make the effort necessary to familiarize themselves with hospital routines and develop friendly relationships with doctors and hospital personnel who are important in the treatment of their patients. They show appreciation for good performance and displeasure with bad.

5. Some doctors manage their patients well, anticipating and conditioning patients and their relatives on the timing of discharge and postdischarge requirements, and provide hospital planning with as much advance notice of impending discharge problems as possible.

In short, the competent well-organized physician who knows *what to do* for a hospitalized patient, *when to do it* and *in what order* has a far more beneficial effect on hospital utilization rates and length of stay in the types of hospitals we visited than regulatory programs can possibly have. With a minimum of extraneous activity, such physicians do what needs to be done, understanding and effectively using the hospital's formal systems and developing their own informal methods to assure that various hospital departments provide them with what they want, when they need it. (An interesting, illustrative case study appears as Appendix 2 on pages 134–36)

The impact of the example provided by such physicians can be very persuasive. It is timely, it is local, and it is something that other physicians can directly observe and emulate. If more physicians do adopt the practice patterns of these leaders, two important things can happen:

1. the informal systems developed by ancillary departments as exceptions for a few physicians can become formalized as standard operating procedures for all physicians, and
2. the overall standards of care within a medical staff can be modified as more and more physicians adopt various aspects of the more innovative care patterns.

It would be unfair to state that during the course of our brief stay at each hospital, we were able to document multiple instances of this type of attitudinal evolution. Nonetheless, several people in various institutions described examples of it.

At one teaching institution we were frequently told how the medical staff and, therefore, the teaching program have become imbued with an attitude that encourages innovation and short length of stay. In another institution, physicians collectively review the procedures used by their colleagues and themselves and exchange suggestions at departmental meetings on methods of practice that might make patient care proceed more smoothly and easily for the individual physician. And in all institutions, inefficiencies that result in excessive lengths of stay under utilization review standards are brought under pressure through that mechanism. It is likely, however, that no one would contest the fact that this barely scratches the surface and that much remains to be done.

MEDICAL OFFICE BUILDINGS

Medical office buildings of substantial size are located on or immediately adjacent to the campus of nine of the hospitals we visited. Four of the buildings are owned by the hospital while, at five hospitals, there are one or more independently owned buildings. Although all types of doctors are extensively represented, most of those located in these office buildings are surgeons or specialists, frequently with a high proportion of referrals, who spend a substantial portion of their time in the hospital. In no case did the buildings provide offices for as many as 25 percent of the doctors on the medical staff.

Proponents of immediately adjacent doctor's offices emphasize:

1. the positive effects of frequent and easy access to a variety of doctors for discussion and formal consultation on patient problems;
2. the opportunity for face-to-face consultations as a supplement to or for written consultation reports;
3. the time-saving features for the patient and the doctor and the opportunity for frequent visits to the hospital as test results are available, crises arise, etc.; and
4. the greater willingness to participate in hospital affairs that arises from easy access to the hospital without loss of transit time, inconvenience, etc.

Those questioning or opposing such offices stress:

1. accessibility to patients throughout the service area — most patients do not require the hospital's services at any one time;
2. the need for patient contact throughout the area if the hospital is to receive patient referrals from the doctor rather than, in effect, have the patient make the choice of hospital on his own initiative;
3. the potential for schism and clique that develops between the "ins" and the "outs";
4. the use of scarce land (if a limiting factor) for both building and parking; and
5. the annoyance of owner-tenant relationships.

Solely from the perspective of this study, one would conclude that the adjacent medical offices would reduce length of stay through increasing the frequency and speed of access of attending physicians to other physicians and to the patient. One would likewise conclude, as will be discussed in Chapter V, that the presence of a substantial number of doctors in a single building — whether adjacent to the hospital or not — might relieve some of the pressure on outpatient hospital services by making it possible to carry them out in well-equipped medical offices. Finally, one would conclude that some of these advantages can be achieved, in part, through medical office buildings that are not adjacent but that are located relatively near to the hospital.

V

Making Appropriate Use of Alternatives to Hospital Care: The Effective Use of Other Community Resources

The extent to which hospital facilities are utilized depends in part on the availability of other alternatives in the community and, in part, on the manner in which the hospital and its actual or potential patients make use of them. This section attempts to discuss only limited aspects of this subject under the following headings:

- The Hospital as Part of the Health Care System
- Doctors as Part of the Health Care System

THE HOSPITAL AS PART OF THE HEALTH CARE SYSTEM

"Health care system" is a term that has been frequently used in recent years. From the perspective of local, state, and federal health-planning agencies, it is viewed primarily as a coordinated stream of services provided by hospitals and a variety of other community health institutions. The efficient system is viewed as one which is not duplicative and contains few, if any, barriers to the movement of patients between the various services. Such a point of view implies that the patient should be treated by the various institutional units in a way that will minimize health care costs, particularly the costs of acute hospital care.

The objective of this study — to find ways to save scarce bed capacity in high-occupancy hospitals for patients who really need acute care — is not inconsistent with the view of a health system set forth above. The basic strategy is:

- to lead the community to reduce illnesses or injuries requiring hospitalization or to find ways to detect and treat them in their preacute stages,
- to divert prospective inpatients to other treatment facilities entirely or for as much as possible of the prehospital and posthospital phases of their illness, and
- to speed up the diagnosis, treatment and recovery of patients during their period of hospitalization.

Table V-1 shows the most significant activities of the health care system from the viewpoint of acute-care hospitals and the agencies or institutions that are most active in carrying them out.

SOME GENERAL OBSERVATIONS

A few generalizations are of interest.

1. Every hospital we visited coordinates its activities with all or virtually all of the agencies or institutions shown in Table V-1, but there are sharp variations in the degree to which this is done.
2. The degree of interest shown by most hospitals in other sectors of the health care system seems to vary in direct proportion to how much and how directly they affect the basic services that the hospital provides. Thus, most hospitals tend to be only marginally involved in preventive medicine and education and various forms of special care and after-recovery community support. However, three of the hospitals we visited (four, including the Kaiser group) are markedly more active in developing or strengthening many elements of the system.
3. Over the years there has been an increasing tendency for hospitals to own and operate agencies that previously were independent entities. This is most notable in the case of home care (or visiting-nurse agencies) where the impetus undoubtedly comes from the hospital's need or desire to discharge patients before they are fully recovered. While the step is a big one, sufficient concern exists over the availability of beds in nursing homes and extended care facilities so that more hospitals may join the few that now operate them. Further

impetus for this move may also be provided by the opportunity that exists in many areas of the country to generate funds for general hospital use.

In the remainder of this chapter, we will comment on some of these matters in more detail.

PREVENTIVE PROGRAMS AND PUBLIC EDUCATION

None of the hospitals has mounted a program that it believes has had an important impact on the lifestyle or early detection of illnesses of the people living in its service area. In most instances, the hospitals make only token efforts — usually as an element of their community relations program — although they recognize (1) that they frequently support more substantial efforts made by national, political, and health organizations (e.g., the Heart Association) and (2) that the medical effects of their own efforts, while small, are still worthwhile. Several reasons are usually given for this:

1. where it has been attempted, the public has taken little more than a casual interest in such programs;
2. hospitals have few sources of funding that will enable them to offer these programs on a sufficiently massive basis to make a significant impression; and,
3. there is often disagreement, both within and without the hospital, about whether this is an appropriate undertaking for an acute-care hospital.

They also note that individual doctors often actively participate in organizations relating to their fields of interest.

Several hospitals contrast with this pattern. One, in particular, has made a major financial and philosophical commitment to preventive and educational programs and at least four hospitals have developed one or more successful programs that appear to be having a limited but worthwhile impact within the communities served. These efforts will be discussed in the balance of this section.

General-community education programs. Most hospitals make available a variety of informational pamphlets and publish articles in local newspapers that reach what they believe is a limited and irregular audience. In addition, they provide speakers for numerous outside organizations and, in recent years, for lectures and half- and full-day conferences

TABLE V-1

I. Preventive Medicine and Public Education
 – Physical examinations in doctors' offices
 – Public education by hospitals; by heart, lung, and similar associations; by public health agencies

II. Diagnosis and Treatment of Patients

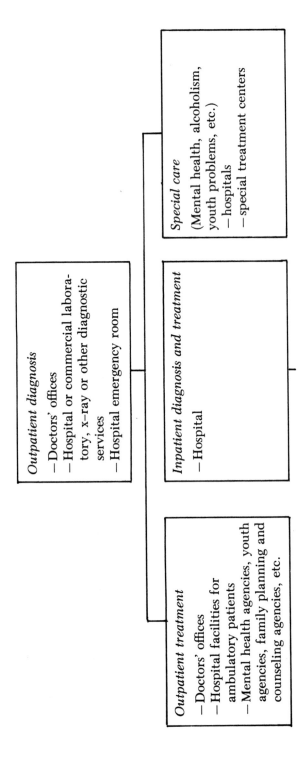

Outpatient diagnosis
 – Doctors' offices
 – Hospital or commercial laboratory, x-ray or other diagnostic services
 – Hospital emergency room

Inpatient diagnosis and treatment
 – Hospital

Special care
(Mental health, alcoholism, youth problems, etc.)
 – hospitals
 – special treatment centers

Outpatient treatment
 – Doctors' offices
 – Hospital facilities for ambulatory patients
 – Mental health agencies, youth agencies, family planning and counseling agencies, etc.

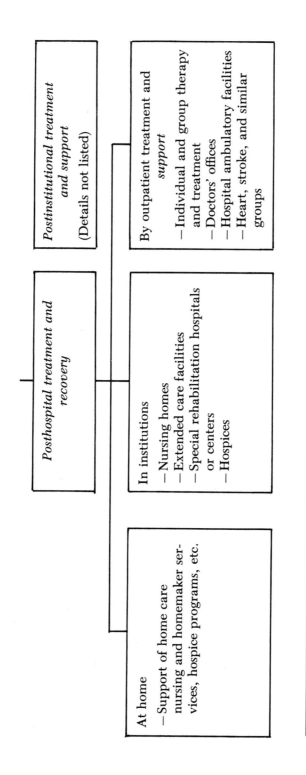

Posthospital treatment and recovery

At home
— Support of home care nursing and homemaker services, hospice programs, etc.

In institutions
— Nursing homes
— Extended care facilities
— Special rehabilitation hospitals or centers
— Hospices

Postinstitutional treatment and support
(Details not listed)

By outpatient treatment and *support*
— Individual and group therapy and treatment
— Doctors' offices
— Hospital ambulatory facilities
— Heart, stroke, and similar groups

to which the public in general or individuals with a special interest in the topic are invited. The major illnesses (e.g., heart, stroke, diabetes, and cancer); social problems such as coping with stress, smoking, and alcoholism; and life-saving techniques such as the Heimlich maneuver and mouth-to-mouth resuscitation are topics which customarily draw a substantial number of people with a direct or indirect personal interest in the topics. Conferences for clergyman on problems such as medical ethics and dealing with dying patients and their families are useful and effective. In recent years, athletic injuries have also been of substantial interest. And, of course, ambulance corps and other emergency personnel are intensely interested in topics bearing on their activities.

One institution in search of both greater reach and impact for its general education programs has taken a particularly innovative approach that combines direct mailings, newspaper articles, and programming on local television. The hospital first mails information about the program (the Health Information Program, or HIP) and a well-labeled folder (called the "HIP Pocket") to households in its service area. Second, it arranges for articles to be written and published in the local daily paper on a regular weekly basis on important medical topics of general interest. And, finally, it arranges for the authors of these articles, usually physicians, to appear on a regularly scheduled television broadcast to discuss a particular subject and answer questions. People are encouraged to clip out the articles and keep them in their "HIP Pocket" for future reference.

TEL-MED. Another program that has achieved broad public participation is the TEL-MED program that is in use at one hospital. TEL-MED involves a library of 200 or more prerecorded messages on health care topics (see Exhibit V-1 for a typical listing of messages). Interested individuals call in and ask for the desired tape by its code number, and the TEL-MED operator plays the tape, approximately one to five minutes in length. Although TEL-MED tape libraries have been installed in a number of hospitals throughout the country, the success of the program is said to vary considerably. In this hospital, 28,300 TEL-MED calls were received in the past eight months. The success of the observed program is in large part attributed to the hospital's decision to mail the descriptive brochures to all of the 60,000 households in the hospital's service area and to follow up with extensive, continuing newspaper publicity. Ongoing operating costs are greatly minimized by the exclusive use of volunteers to staff the TEL-MED program.

Wellness program. The most ambitious undertaking by any hospital we visited was the creation of a "wellness program" at one western hospital.

EXHIBIT V-1

TEL-MED BROCHURE

TEL-MED is

a special collection of health information tapes prepared by professionals to help you and your family:

- know more about your own health
- recognize early signs of illness
- STAY HEALTHY!

TEL-MED is a free service
funded and staffed by
The Valley Hospital Auxiliary.

TEL-MED tapes are

- easy to understand
- 1 to 5 minutes long
- as close and as private as your telephone.

All tapes listed have been reviewed and approved by the Medical Society of New Jersey and The Valley Hospital Medical Staff.

To use TEL-MED

just call the phone number shown in this booklet. When the operator answers, give the number of the tape you want to hear. Calls are automatically disconnected at the end of each tape.

TEL-MED is not to be used

- in an emergency
- to decide if you have a health problem
- to replace your doctor.

Only qualified professionals are equipped to diagnose and treat medical problems.

**TEL-MED is for you.
Use it as often as you like.**

TEL-MED Tape Library
Always ask for tapes by number.

Aging
86 Old Age Freckles: Dangerous?
144 Emotional Experiences Of Dying
155 Medicare
173 Menopause
175 Fears Of The After-Forty Man
474 Reading Glasses & Presbyopia

Arthritis & Rheumatism
126 Gout
128 Rheumatoid Arthritis
129 Bursitis
131 Arthritis & Quackery
1037 Plastic Surgery for Rheumatoid Arthritis of the Hands

Birth Control
53 Vasectomy
54 Tubal Ligation
55 The Pill
56 Intrauterine Devices
57 The Rhythm Method
58 Diaphragm, Foam & Condom

Blood & Circulation
25 Hypertension & Blood Pressure
29 Atherosclerosis & Blood Pressure
34 Anemia
566 Sickle Cell Anemia

Cancer
6 Breast Cancer
176 Cancer Of The Prostate Gland
177 Cancer Services & Rehabilitation
178 Breast Cancer Rehabilitation
179 Lung Cancer
180 Cancer Of The Colon & Rectum
181 Cancer: The Curable Disease
183 Cancer: Seven Warning Signals
184 Hodgkin's Disease
185 Cancer Of The Skin
186 Uterine Cancer
187 Drugs That Treat Cancer
188 Radiation Therapy For Cancer
190 Thyroid Cancer
192 Leukemia
520 Bone Cancer
521 Bladder Cancer
522 Brain Cancer
523 Larynx Cancer
524 Mouth Cancer
525 Stomach Cancer

Children: Infants to Teens
3 Medicine Poisoning & Your Child
18 Tonsillectomy
20 Rheumatic Fever
48 Thumb Sucking
49 No No: What It Means To Toddlers
50 Teens: The Rebellious Years
51 When A New Baby Creates Jealousy
62 The Premature Baby
71 Aspirin For Children
73 Earache In Children
75 Pinworms
81 Nervous Tics In Children
133 Advice For Parents Of Teenagers
220 Limping In Children
224 Mumps
225 Croup
226 Should My Child Stay Home Today?
227 Measles
229 Chickenpox
230 Cleft Lip & Palate
231 Hearing Loss In Children
232 Speech Problems In Children
233 Diabetes In Children
235 Large & Protruding Ears
236 Cystic Fibrosis
237 Whooping Cough
238 Hiccups
239 Necessary Inoculations
260 Supplies For The Newborn
261 Care Of The Newborn
262 Sudden Infant Death
263 Teething
310 Baby Teeth
381 Muscular Dystrophy In Children
400 Tommy Gets His Tonsils Out
401 Personal Hygiene For A Child
402 Where Did I Come From, Mama?
403 Young Child's Eating & Meals
404 Brothers & Sisters Getting Along
405 The Single Parent Family
406 Accidents, Safety & Children
408 Discipline & Punishment
431 Child Protective Services
433 Foster Care of Children
471 Children's Vision
1082 Sports Tips For Youngsters
1083 Little League Elbow
5004 Children and Death
5005 Reye's Syndrome

Dental & Mouth Care
301 Flossing Your Teeth
302 Brushing Teeth Effectively
303 Dental Plaque
304 Diet Tips For Dental Health
305 Malocclusion: Crooked Teeth
306 Wisdom Teeth
307 Gum Disease: Warning Signs
308 Replacing Teeth: When & Why
309 Canker Sores & Fever Blisters
311 Toothache: What Not To Do
312 Abscessed Teeth Can Be Saved
313 Dentures: Food For Thought
314 Bad Breath: What Causes It
315 Dental X-Rays: Really Necessary?
317 Dental Insurance
318 Reducing Dental Costs
319 How To Select A Dentist
321 Which Toothpaste?
323 Are You Afraid Of The Dentist?

Diabetes & Hypoglycemia
11 Diabetes: What Are The Signs?
22 Foot Care For Diabetics
565 Hypoglycemia
609 Diabetic Diets

Diet
600 Cholesterol In Your Diet
601 Low Soft Diet
602 How Important are Trace Minerals in Your diet?
603 Breakfast: Why Is It Important?
604 A Guide To Good Eating
605 Food Stamps & Good Nutrition
608 Snacks

Digestive System
2 What Is A "Normal" Bowel?
44 Hemorrhoids
44 Ulcers
45 Indigestion
78 Appendicitis
196 Peptic Ulcers
198 Hiatal Hernia
199 Colitis & Bowel Disorders
219 Laxatives
630 Diarrhea
631 Gall Bladder Trouble
662 Diverticulosis; Diverticulitis

Drug & Alcohol Abuse
134 LSD
136 Amphetamines & Barbiturates
137 Marijuana
138 Narcotics
942 Alcoholism: Scope Of The Problem
943 Is Drinking A Problem?
945 So You Love An Alcoholic
946 How AA Can Help Problem Drinkers
1222 Drug Abuse Resources in Bergen County

Eye Care
9 Glaucoma
470 Seeing Spots & Floaters
472 Cataracts
473 Contact Lenses: A Closer Look
474 Reading Glasses & Presbyopia
1216 Using Eye Drops

First Aid
91 Severe Bleeding
93 Electrical Shock
94 Shock
96 Poisoning By Mouth
98 Head Injuries
99 Sprains
101 Burns

EXHIBIT V-1, *continued*

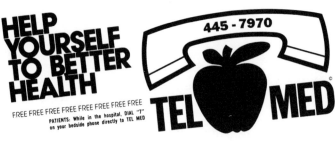

HELP YOURSELF TO BETTER HEALTH

445-7970

TEL MED

FREE FREE FREE FREE FREE FREE FREE FREE
PATIENTS: While in the hospital, DIAL "7" on your bedside phone directly to TEL MED

Patients: Dial "7"

Monday through Friday:
10 a.m.-3 p.m.
7 p.m.-9 p.m.

Saturday, Sunday and Holidays:
1 p.m.-4 p.m.

A community service of

The Valley Hospital Auxiliary
Ridgewood, N.J. 07451

General
- 107 Suspected Heart Attack
- 108 Fainting
- 109 Epileptic Convulsions
- 111 Choking
- 118 Animal Bites
- 121 Bee Stings
- 1031 Cuts & Skin Lacerations

- 429 What Is Tel-Med?
- 17 Lockjaw
- 19 Cut Your Medical Costs Nine Ways
- 26 Stroke & Apoplexy
- 35 Headaches
- 36 Hiccups
- 37 Backaches
- 40 Viruses: What Are They?
- 41 Skiing Season: Getting Ready
- 42 I'm Just Tired, Doctor
- 46 Lumps & Bumps Of Arms & Legs
- 59 Blood Transfusion Blood Bank
- 84 Dizziness
- 125 Epilepsy
- 139 Help Yourself Get Well
- 140 How Safe are Drugs?
- 141 How New Drugs are Tested
- 150 New Jersey Temporary Disability
- 154 Medicaid
- 162 Hepatitis
- 174 Masturbation
- 191 Varicose Veins
- 193 Baldness & Falling Hair
- 194 What Happens When A Disc Slips
- 195 Bee Sting: It Can Cause Death
- 201 Neck Pains
- 430 About Medical Insurance
- 726 Psychosomatic Illness
- 825 Multiple Sclerosis
- 969 Infectious Mononucleosis
- 1081 Health Hints For Campers
- 1101 Exercising: Warm Up Slowly
- 1215 Frostbite
- 5000 This Is Your Valley Hospital Auxiliary
- 5001 Hospitalization Insurance - Utilization Review
- 5002 Living Through Grief
- 5003 Constructive Grief Management
- 5006 Meals on Wheels
- 5007 Valley Hospital Patient Bill of Rights
- 5008 The Society of The Valley Hospital Runners
- 5009 How To Avoid Heart Stroke

Speech & Hearing
- 43 Stuttering & Other Speech Defects
- 76 Otosclerosis & Hearing Loss
- 450 From Hearing Loss to Hearing Aid
- 451 Hearing Loss From Noise

Heart
- 21 Cigarettes & Heart Disease
- 23 Diet & Heart Disease
- 27 Health & Heart Checkups
- 28 Reducing Risk Of Heart Attack
- 30 Angina Pectoris
- 63 Early Warning Of Heart Attack
- 65 Chest Pains
- 72 Heart Failure

Home Health Care
- 10 Poisons In The Home
- 60 Power Lawn Mower Dangers
- 61 Fever: What Does It Mean?
- 89 Treatment Using Cold
- 160 Cockroaches
- 164 Your Family Health
- 165 Home Care For The Bedridden
- 166 Medical Supplies For The Home
- 167 Exercise For The Bedridden
- 168 Taking Pulse, Temp & Respiration
- 171 Prescription Medicine

Mental Health
- 33 Tension
- 159 Hypnosis
- 432 Upset Emotionally? Help Available
- 727 Schizophrenia
- 728 When Should I See A Psychiatrist?

Pregnancy
- 5 Early Prenatal Care
- 12 Am I Really Pregnant?
- 67 Warning Signs In Pregnancy

Respiratory System
- 7 Pneumonia
- 13 Pulmonary Emphysema
- 38 Influenza
- 90 Hay Fever
- 576 Bronchial Asthma
- 581 Chronic Cough
- 582 Shortness Of Breath

Skin & Plastic Surgery
- 79 Dandruff
- 80 Ringworm
- 82 Psoriasis: Why The Mystery?
- 83 Impetigo
- 124 Shingles
- 172 Acne
- 235 Large & Protruding Ears
- 518 Itching Skin
- 1032 Blepharoplasty For Baggy Eyelids
- 1033 Otoplasty For Misshapen Ears
- 1034 What Is Plastic Surgery?
- 1035 Abdominoplasty For Stomach Lifts
- 1036 Cosmetic Body Surgery
- 1038 Microsurgery and Replacement of Amputated Parts
- 1040 Plastic Surgery
- 1041 Rhinoplasty
- 1042 Hair Transplants
- 1043 Chemical Skin Peeling
- 1044 Plastic Surgery for Scars

- 68 Infertility
- 69 Artificial Insemination
- 881 Breast Feeding Your Baby
- 882 Emotions After Childbirth
- 883 Caring For Yourself After A Baby

Smoking
- 693 Weight Control While Quitting
- 694 Why A Woman Should Quit Smoking
- 695 Reducing Risks Of Smoking
- 696 How Smoking Affects Your Health
- 697 Do You Want To Quit Smoking?
- 698 When Do You Get Out Of Smoking?
- 699 What Do You Gain By Quitting Smoking?
- 700 Effects Of Smoking On Nonsmokers

Urinary Tract
- 77 Kidney Stones
- 1140 Blood In The Urine
- 1141 Kidney & Urinary Tract Infections

Venereal Disease
- 8 Venereal Disease
- 15 Syphilis
- 16 Gonorrhea

Women
- 31 Vaginitis
- 32 Unwanted Pregnancy
- 74 Why A D&C?
- 182 What Is A Pap Test?
- 889 Hysterectomy
- 1030 Cosmetic Surgery Of The Breasts

In its Statement of Mission, this institution affirms its belief that the ultimate objective of all health and medical service is promotion of the improved health status of individuals. To further this objective, this institution began a wellness program in April, 1978. The initial pilot program, conducted with 100 employees and/or their spouses, emphasized nutrition, stress management, and physical fitness. The objective was simple — to increase individual awareness of the benefits of a "wellness lifestyle." Individual participants were responsible for establishing and fulfilling their own program. Following a successful pilot program, this hospital has expanded the program, offering it to all employees and physicians, as well as their families, and to members of a number of civic and youth groups. Other hospitals in the area have expressed considerable interest in this program and the "wellness" concept.

Screening programs. We were somewhat surprised to find such a limited use of general and specific screening programs, executive physical examinations, and other large-scale detection programs among the hospitals we visited. Except at one or two institutions, there appears to be a general consensus that screening programs achieve very limited results unless they are aimed directly at a specific, high-risk category of individuals.

The successful screening programs appear to have achieved this result because of a particularly supportive group of physicians or massive community support. They deal with a very specific topic and are held at times and places that encourage broad support. Rather than being "one-shot deals," they tend to be held frequently and are well-published as part of an ongoing effort.

Parent education. One western hospital has established a parent-education department, offering the community a variety of classes designed "to enhance the quality of life as it relates to self and one's relationships with family, spouse and friends." Courses are offered at various times throughout the year at a very minimal charge. Although many of the instructors are hospital employees, the hospital contracts with specialists outside the hospital to provide the instruction in specific classes. Course offerings include:

1. Prenatal classes — for expectant parents
2. Adapting to Adopting — for couples anticipating adopting
3. Marriage-Go-Round — for couples anticipating marriage or desiring to enrich their relationship
4. Gynecological Surgery — for patients facing gynecological surgery and members of their families

5. Show and Share — for parents of infants, ages one week through one year
6. The Preschool Class — for parents of children, ages one through four
7. The School-Age Child
8. The Adolescence Class
9. The Middle Adult Years
10. The Maturity Class — for persons in the retirement years
11. Singleness in the 1970s

While this program operates at a deficit, the loss is modest. The institution is convinced that the value of the program to the community more than justifies the cost.

Developing and Working with Other Units of the Health Care System

Since many of the activities and elements of the health care system have already been commented on extensively, the present discussion will, for the most part, focus on matters that are not covered elsewhere in this book.

Physicians' office buildings. A substantial portion of the doctors at each of the hospitals that we visited practices out of a medical office building that contains from about 5 to 50 other doctors. In some instances, there is no professional relationship among the doctors; often, however, a relationship does exist in one of a variety of formal and informal arrangements. At times, the office building is on or immediately adjacent to the hospital campus, but often it is a more substantial distance away, depending upon the distribution of population throughout the service area. In rural areas, a distance of ten or more miles might be involved. At times, the building is owned by the hospital, the doctors, an HMO-type corporation, or an independent investor — but this is unimportant. What seems to be evident from our study is that, in two sets of circumstances, hospitals are taking the initiative in treating the office building as part of the health care system and, in a third instance, the doctors are doing so.

Several hospitals are establishing or subsidizing an office for one or more doctors in rural areas that is better equipped than can probably be justified by the economics of the practice. This office is being provided, as of the moment, in order to provide health care that is currently needed, but also with an eye to the probable growth in population in coming years.

The second extension involves the expansion of the range of diagnostic services available in the doctors' offices. At times, these are being carried out completely by equipment in the medical office building, but more often the patients are sent to the hospital or a commercial facility, or — to come to the point of interest — a few hospitals that we visited are contracting to provide laboratory and x-ray services to the doctors, usually by using some equipment located in the medical offices, but carrying out the bulk of the analysis and interpretation in the hospital.

Finally, well-equipped medical offices are — especially, but not necessarily, in HMO-types of situations — becoming a combination of doctors' offices and clinics, rendering not only diagnostic services and the types of care normally associated with doctors' offices but also moving incrementally into "lumps and bumps" removal and other types of work normally thought of as being at the lower end of hospital care.

Home care and "homemaker" services. As has been previously discussed, many hospitals are intensely interested in the quality of the home care services available to hospitalized patients who cannot be discharged without this type of assistance, except to a nursing home. In many cities, the quality and availability of care provided by independent visiting-nurse associations are excellent. Their acceptance by the medical staff and their coordination with discharge-planning personnel result in a productive and satisfactory relationship. Complete coverage is provided for a variety of patients, from new mothers to the elderly.

Five other hospitals are not satisfied with respect to one or more of the four criteria for home care — quality of care, coverage, coordination, and acceptance. Therefore, they have established their own service as a department of the hospital or as a quasi-independent entity, and they are very pleased with the results. Acceptance by doctors in particular, has been said to have improved greatly as a result of the more frequent personal contacts and association with the hospital-based staff. Two of the hospitals have aggressively promoted this service, not only by providing it to other hospitals but also by providing it under contract to a number of municipalities.

Most hospitals find that a number of patients can also benefit from a "homemaker" service that assists with shopping and nonmedical requirements within the home, delivers a hot meal to the home daily, or helps out in some other manner. All of the hospitals use existing community resources for this purpose.

Nursing homes and extended care facilities. Nursing homes and extended care facilities are undoubtedly the most important components of the health care system with which the hospital must deal. When they are available, as is most often the case, they facilitate the rapid movement of the patient through the system according to need. But, when nursing-home and extended-care-facility beds are not available — as is often the case in some states — hospitals are forced to retain the patients. The principal culprit is undoubtedly at the Medicaid-reimbursement level, but there are a lot of other difficulties as varied as nursing home scandals and long-outstanding Certificates of Need for new beds on which progress is proceeding very slowly.

Most of the hospitals rely on nursing and extended care facilities owned and operated by others. However, two hospitals have taken the opposite position in states where the reimbursement system permits some flexibility. One is developing a motel-like facility to handle a portion of its patients, while the second has acquired nursing homes with a bed capacity substantially in excess of its needs. It is our impression that the managerial aspects of nursing-home operations are greatly simplified by factors such as long lengths of stay and waiting lists for admission and that, with reasonable reimbursement, there may be an important role for the hospital to play here — especially with regard to the difficult patient who cannot benefit from sophisticated hospital care but is too ill to be suitable for most nursing home settings.

Rehabilitation centers. Three of the hospitals surveyed have an independent inpatient-rehabilitation unit. Two of them (averaging 25 beds) are on-campus and attached to the main hospitals, while the third is located off-site with 44 beds. A fourth institution made a portion of its campus available to an independent, specialized, and sophisticated rehabilitation hospital with 80 beds. All are satisfied that these are highly beneficial additions to the hospital's regular acute-care services. The major benefits of these units to the "mother" hospital appear to be the following:

1. They permit the hospital to free acute-care beds more quickly since, after stabilization in an acute-care bed, patients requiring rehabilitation care can promptly be transferred to the rehabilition unit.
2. Because of the ready availability of skilled rehabilitation personnel, including a medical director, patients who are in the main hospital for a debilitating injury, stroke, etc., may begin an appropriate course of therapy more quickly.
3. They may present an opportunity to increase total bed capacity, since the addition of rehabilitation beds may be more attractive than medical/surgical beds to HSAs and other regulatory agencies.

Another institution, which does not have its own rehabilitation unit, has a formal arrangement with a county facility specializing in rehabilitation care and other long-term patients. The county facility has a full-time staff of six general practitioners, supplemented by a significant number of attending physicians, most of whom are also on the staff of the hospital. Accordingly, most physicians have the choice of following up on a patient at the county facility or of referring that patient to a physician with whom they are familiar.

Alcoholism centers. Three of the hospitals we visited have inpatient alcoholism treatment centers, all of which are of recent origin. Several others have such centers under study, recognizing the magnitude of the problem and the nature of the role that the hospital can perform during the two to four weeks the patient is in the hospital as part of the total treatment program.

The typical alcoholism center of a hospital receives, after detoxification, patients who have voluntarily decided to enter the program. During a period of approximately two weeks while the patient is in the hospital, he or she and, usually, mother, father, and/or spouse receive extensive psychological support and therapy; education about the physiological impacts of alcohol; and, of course, good meals (and a period of abstinence from liquor). The patient upon discharge usually receives a limited amount of posthospital counseling from the alcoholism center extending over the next year or two, but primary reliance for this service is placed on the activities of the local chapter of Alcoholics Anonymous. Similar organizations are also available for close relatives, many of whom participate in these activities.

The hospitals with such programs are both enthusiastic about them and aware of the complexity of the basic problem. They are pleased that this service is increasingly recognized as reimbursable under various Blue Cross and private insurance plans.

Hospice programs. The development of hospice programs to care for terminally ill, usually cancerous patients has received considerable attention in the past two years. Nationwide, a small number of hospitals have established hospice programs, including two of the hospitals we visited. On the basis of very preliminary results, they indicate satisfaction from both a medical and a humanitarian standpoint and recognize that, at the same time, the hospice program represents an efficient use of the health care system, that has freed a number of beds for other patients.

In two hospitals, the program involves having the patient remain in his or her own home and supporting the patient and family with special training, extensive volunteer support, and adequate assistance by visiting nurses and the attending physician.

Posthospital therapeutic activities. A number of community agencies, usually with encouragement but not financial support from the hospital, are developing and carrying out therapeutic support services for previously hospitalized patients. These services primarily relate to:

1. alcoholism
2. cardiac rehabilitation, and
3. stroke.

Individual hospital programs. Somehow, this discussion of individual agencies and institutions does not properly indicate the degree of commitment by certain individual hospitals to participation in an overall health system. Most hospitals are relatively active with respect to at least a few of the components of health systems that we have mentioned. Two hospitals, however, are far more heavily committed than the others. One, whose commitment is fundamentally philosophical, owns and operates two satellite emergency life-support units on the periphery of their service area (using paramedics and radio communication), a gerontology center, a wellness program, a major community health education program, and a motel-like facility for the families of inpatients. They have also developed a residential facility and program for the elderly.

The other hospital, whose motives appear to be a mixture of both financial and philosophical desirability, is actively involved with the development of a program which will offer subscribers a full spectrum of care — from outpatient services to extended nursing-home care. The institution currently operates its own visiting-nurse service (which also provides physical therapy services) and, through a separate corporate structure, it also operates nursing homes.

DOCTORS AS PART OF THE THE HEALTH CARE SYSTEM

Virtually every organizational form of medical practice — formal and informal — exists in the hospitals and cities that we visited. However, if one looks past the economic and organizational differences, it becomes clear that all doctors are involved in some form of group practice in which they are increasingly dependent on each other and the institutions that serve them, not only for medical skills but also for speed of access and extent of coverage. Whether, as individuals, they are sole practitioners, members of single multi-specialty groups, Individual Practice Associations (IPAs), or HMOs is by all odds of secondary importance.

All of the hospitals we visited emphasize the importance of the formal organization and activities of the medical staff, medical board, and medical departments as well as the necessity for strong committed leadership. They likewise underscore the necessity of obtaining substantial physician input and participation in the development of policy and key managerial decisions. And they stress the need for and the enormous productive value to physicians and hospitals of a strong collegial relationship among the physicians themselves.

The Doctor as Patient Manager

One of the doctor's roles as patient manager is to select the component of the health care system that best matches the patient's needs and to choose the time at which the patient should move from one component to the other. This requires an understanding of both the capabilities of these components and their costs, if "best" is to represent an appropriate trade-off of medical benefits and financial consequences. And, finally, the doctor must make an effort to help the patient find his way through and adapt to the system.

IPAs and HMOs

We did not note important differences in physicians' managerial performance, based on whether they are solo or group practitioners. There is, of course, a noticeable difference when physicians are organized into HMOs or IPAs. The implications of these types of physician organizations are well known and will not be repeated here.

One or more HMOs or IPAs is in existence in about half of the cities in which the hospitals we visited are located. In most cases, these came into being without the direct involvement or support of the hospitals. However, in some situations, the indirect involvement or support of the hospital was of critical importance. In fact, one hospital is currently providing the direct impetus for the development of an IPA.

Regardless of the hospital's role in the development of these organizations, their ongoing relationship is critical. On the one hand, the hospital has an organized and coordinated group with which to work, and communications about services, use rates, and physician needs can be accomplished directly and effectively. On the other hand, as has been mentioned, the cost of hospital services is of greater interest to physicians, and physicians become more careful, more sophisticated consumers of health care. In every instance, the hospitals find that their common interests far exceed their differences and that the relationship tends both to keep them on their toes and to be satisfactory.

VI

Informing,
Influencing, and Adapting
to the Hospital's Environment

While the rate of occupancy and length of stay are, in themselves, terms of little difficulty, they are the end-products of ideas, actions, and relationships of substantial medical, physical, administrative, and financial complexity. Informing, influencing, and adapting to the hospital's environment with respect to rate of occupancy and length of stay must reflect, of necessity, this complexity. However, these efforts must also reflect the need and capacity of a hospital to absorb the diverse publics that make up its environment — the medical staff, the general public, patients and concerned relatives, and regulatory and reimbursing agencies.

It might have been well if we had devoted a greater portion of our interviews to this subject. However, we did not and probably we would have found that we lacked the sophisticated knowledge of communications techniques necessary to understand and evaluate what we saw and heard, anyway. Nevertheless, we believe it may be valuable to pass on a number of the impressions we received at various hospitals.

THE MEDICAL STAFF — THE MOST IMPORTANT PUBLIC

1. The medical staff is, in most respects, the hospital's most important public (a) because it initiates so many actions that directly affect the occupancy and length of stay and (b) because it so heavily influences the attitudes of patients and concerned relatives.

2. While all doctors respond to situations that are clear-cut and visible, their understanding of the reasons for them varies tremendously. Most doctors are flexible and cooperative in their responses and, like the rest of us, seek out the paths that will accommodate them with the least difficulty. The range of possibilities they consider tends to progress incrementally from what they consider normal practice. Once a problem — e.g., bed shortages — exists for a considerable period of time, the behavior patterns it fosters will be considered normal.

3. Physicians differ widely in the nature of their practices, their position in the medical staff hierarchy, their participation in medical staff activities, the length of time they have been on the staff, and in other respects. The knowledge they have of hospital operations, procedures, and strategies differs similarly — substantially more than it would among leaders in most large organizations.

4. Because of these differences — and because doctors seem inherently to look primarily to other doctors for knowledge and advice — the knowledge and opinions of the formal and informal leaders of the medical staff are crucial. So is their personal example.

5. A general exposure of the entire staff to matters affecting occupancy and length of stay and to the impact that their actions and decisions have on these matters is undoubtedly useful. So are the reminders (liked or disliked) provided by the general presence of utilization review and similar personnel, the specific cases with which individual physicians are forced to deal, and the discussions of these topics at departmental meetings.

6. At some point, the amount of information that can be transmitted in a more or less passive fashion drops off. Understanding then jumps enormously with constructive participation in the process of identifying, studying, and deciding what to do about overall and specific problems. Fortunately, this participation improves the quality of the solutions and the backing they will receive upon implementation. It also helps to establish the points and ways in which the hospital should adapt to the doctor, as well as the reverse.

Participation is normally associated with doctors at or near the top of the medical staff hierarchy. Several hospitals had physicians with full voting rights on the board of trustees and additional physicians on board committees. At another hospital, physicians constitute 130 of the 200 voting members of the hospital corporation. And, finally, of course, the medical staff of all hospitals have their own committee organizations to deal with at least selected aspects of these problems.

As several hospitals have demonstrated, participation can also be very effective at the departmental level, both in gaining understanding and developing practical solutions. In meetings at that level, all doctors are expected to participate.

7. Statistical data, summarized and organized in a fashion that facilitates understanding and use can be very effective not only in providing dimension to a problem or opportunity but also in demonstrating the reality of its existence in a manner that words cannot do. Most doctors are very skillful in working with numbers.

8. Positive incentives — especially peer approval — are very effective and preferable to the alternative. It is, however, wishful thinking to believe that all doctors will respond sufficiently to these incentives and, thus, disincentives are also essential.

THE GENERAL PUBLIC — AN ELUSIVE CONSTITUENCY

1. The general public has a limited — one might almost say a subliminal — interest in occupancy and length of stay until individuals and their "concerned others" are faced with an illness requiring hospitalization.

2. Efforts that are most productive are generally aimed at creating a general awareness in or preconditioning of the individual. In some respects, word-of-mouth communication will suffice. But newspaper articles and other more direct techniques are usually valuable. The extent of this conditioning can be impressive, as in one community where a very high rate of cancellation of elective cases is accepted as normal. One of the more useful results of providing such information is that it helps to prepare patients and relatives for the fact that their length of stay will probably be far shorter than they may have expected or remembered it to be and gives relatives advance notice of the need to prepare for the patient's return.

3. Information relating to ambulatory services and alternatives to inpatient care can be directly productive in reducing inpatient admissions.

4. A judicious and limited distribution of information about controls placed on the hospital by third parties may be important in developing community understanding.

5. Occupancy and length-of-stay information may be important as-

pects of efforts to expand, to raise funds, or to further other hospital objectives. The information provided in those circumstances will reflect the overall design of the information campaign. Rarely, however, will this information be in conflict with information provided to the general public for the purposes described in points 1–4 above.

PATIENTS AND CONCERNED RELATIVES

1. The crucial source of information is the patient's doctor, whose judgment as to choice of hospital, time of admission, and length of stay will normally be accepted by both patient and relatives. General hospital pamphlets can be useful, but they require interpretation for the individual patient in light of that patient's probable experience.
2. Some doctors do an excellent job in preparing the prospective patient and relatives. Others do a poor job, with the bulk falling in between.
3. The hospital's community health services (or discharge planning) personnel are often very useful. There often would be a substantial advantage to bringing them into troublesome situations at an earlier date than is usual — even in advance of admission.

REGULATORY AND REIMBURSING AGENCIES

1. The nature, extent, and rigidity of planning, operating, and financial controls of regulatory agencies and reimbursing organizations make them extremely important elements in the health care field in general as well as in the operation of the individual hospital. Often local governing bodies are also of crucial importance because of their control of zoning.
2. None of the visited hospitals passively accepts all the rules and regulations of these agencies, but the nature and extent of the hospitals' efforts to influence them and the organizations they use for this purpose vary considerably.
3. Some hospitals try to influence and help to administer specific regulations by becoming part of "the establishment." Some hospital employees are voting members of decision-making state or HSA boards and agencies. In fact, the associate director of one hospital is president of the HSA board of trustees and another recently served on a state board that approved major capital projects. A more common position, however, is as a member of an advisory committee with continuing status or a specific short-term mission. Some hospitals

also offer their institutions as guinea pigs in experiments in reimbursements, alternative approaches to medical care, etc.

4. Hospitals also attempt to influence rules and regulations by opposing and counterproposing. They do so, in part, through national and state organizations — normally when all hospitals have interests in common. But often hospitals find that their interests are different from those of other hospitals in the country, in the state, and even in the relatively small area they cover. Thus they find themselves drawn into devoting an increasing part of their time and energy to informing and influencing decisions in directions that they consider appropriate. Most hospitals use a mixture of formal and informal, institutional and personal, and positive and negative approaches, differing mainly in the proportion of each used. Likewise, they differ in the levels they attempt to reach, with some being active all the way to the national level of government and with the major executives of the agencies with which they deal as well as with key staff personnel. Hospitals seem to differ in the extent to which they attempt to inform others of plans in advance of actions. And, finally, they differ in the extent to which they involve doctors, trustees, and influential members of the community in their efforts.

5. Hospitals seem to agree that key issues of current concern, with important implications for occupancy and length of stay, include the following:

   a. adequate reimbursement coverage for alternatives to inpatient care, e.g., for nursing homes, posthospital home care, ambulatory surgery and preadmission or postdischarge testing and therapy;

   b. reimbursement systems that provide incentives for efficiency and reductions in length of stay and that, in fact, do not penalize short lengths of stay, ambulatory care, etc., through an inadequate recognition of cost effects;

   c. reimbursement policies and controls that focus excessively on individual actions and cost centers to the detriment of the effectiveness of the hospital as a whole;

   d. limitations on bed expansion that may be appropriate for a broad area but are inappropriate for an individual hospital; and

   e. zoning problems.

6. All hospitals acknowledge that their efforts to influence regulatory agencies and reimbursement organizations are somewhere between slightly and partially successful on an overall basis and that adaptation is an important element of hospital life.

VII

Census Control
Through Medical Staff
Regulation and Limitation

THE VALLEY HOSPITAL'S SITUATION

At The Valley Hospital, a rapid increase in the size of the active medical staff (up from 183 physicians in 1972 to 254 in 1978) combined with severe limitations on physical expansion of the hospital to create problems of high occupancy and raise serious questions about the hospital's ability to continue its historic policy of accepting unlimited additions to its medical staff. While it was recognized that a hospital's activity is affected by factors other than the size of the medical staff, there was statistical evidence — extending over a number of years — of a direct correlation between the number of admissions and the number of doctors, and between the number of operations and the number of surgeons. A crisis ensued when we were advised that a number of important physicians at a neighboring hospital (close enough so that many of their patients would have followed them) intended to apply for admission at Valley.

After prolonged consideration of the problem, the board of trustees and the medical staff agreed to impose a limitation on further admissions to the medical staff under a procedure that was designed:

1. to be equitable,
2. to discourage the lateral transfer of established physicians from nearby hospitals to Valley, and
3. to continue to encourage the influx of new, young physicians and the introduction of new specialties to the medical staff.

The limitation is worded in the following manner:

> In addition to the requirements for admission to the Active Medical Staff set
> forth in the By-Laws of the Medical Staff..., no person shall be eligible for
> appointment to the Active Medical Staff...with admitting privileges unless
> such person (a) maintains an office within the primary service area, and (b)
> has not been in private practice in...[the four surrounding] Counties for
> more than two years immediately preceding the date of his application, ex-
> cept that neither clause (a) nor clause (b) shall apply to a person whose
> limited specialty is one for which there is a previously determined need in the
> Hospital....As used...[here] "private practice" means maintaining an
> office which is open at regular hours....

We recognized that such a policy might, in the long run, be inadequate to
keep medical-staff size and capacity in balance since the medical staff
would continue to grow, but we hoped to hold it within manageable proportions while searching for a more permanent solution to the problem.

OTHER METHODS OF LIMITING STAFF SIZE

Thus, a primary objective of this study was to identify other mechanisms that have successfully been employed to control the number of
admitting physicians and, thereby, the number of admissions to the hospital. Our success in this endeavor was somewhat limited:

1. We had hoped to find a hospital that had developed and employed a
   "table of organization" for the medical staff, enumerating the pro-
   portionate breakdown of the medical specialties: (For example: per
   100,000 population served, 30 internists, 5 ophthalmologists, 3 urol-
   ogists, etc.). We found none among our study's hospitals, and we
   were unable to locate any hospital in the country using such a system. We were told by the Kaiser group that such a table of organization develops informally at each of its hospitals but that it varies significantly among their hospitals. They further stated that the
   problem is complicated by the lack of correlation between specialty
   title and actual practice that often exists.
2. One hospital has developed for their credentials committee a
   "Numerical Evaluation System" that permits members of the committee to assign points to an applicant in four categories:
   a. Recommendations and references
   b. Training and experience
   c. Communication skills
   d. Identification with the community
   In each category, the applicant may receive between one and four

points. Points for the four categories are accumulated, and the total score given by each member of the Credentials Committee are averaged. Based upon the applicant's specialty and the hospital's need for that specialty, various *minimum* average scores must be attained.

a. An average of 10.0 is required for "Surgeons and Internists whose knowledge and skill are urgently needed."

b. An average of 12.0 is required for "Surgeons and Internists whose knowledge and skills are already possessed in adequate number by members of the Medical Staff (or) all other practitioners other than Surgeons or Internists."

c. An average of 14.0 is required for "Surgeons and Internists whose knowledge and skills are already possessed in abundance by members of the Medical staff."

This procedure has been successfully employed without legal challenge for more than two years. While its most important effect is to upgrade the quality of the staff, it serves to limit growth by the exclusion of those who are unable to meet these criteria.

3. Another hospital with very high occupancy has maintained a moratorium on medical staff growth for the past two years — a moratorium which has successfully withstood a court challenge. At this hospital, the only new physicians permitted to join the active staff are those who replace members who have resigned, retired, or died, and who meet the following criteria:

a. they have a beneficial impact on the hospital (i.e., by adding a particular specialty or talent), and

b. they do not have a negative effect on the overall availability of beds.

Since most physicians in this area are in single-specialty group practices, the most likely candidates are physicians who have joined a group to replace a previous member or are highly qualified in new subspecialties.

The hospital has taken great care to follow legally correct, formal procedures in reviewing applications for staff membership. Further, in 1978, it successfully defended a suit by two otolaryngologists who sought staff privileges on the basis that hospitals in other areas did not possess adequate facilities or staff for the performance of certain surgical procedures. The hospital effectively demonstrated that a denial of privileges to these physicians did not cause undue hardship to them because, in fact, the staff and facilities of the neighboring institution were adequate.

People at this hospital readily agreed that the impacts of this staff moratorium have not all been positive. The board of trustees and

the administration expressed concern about:
a. the number of good residents that have left the area because of an inability to join this staff promptly, and
b. the quasi-dual admission procedure occasioned by the fact that doctors joining existing groups normally are those most likely to be admitted.
However, they believe continuation of the procedure is essential to the welfare of the hospital.
4. Elsewhere, we found situations where gradations of medical staff privileges exist. However, with the exception of one institution where new physicians are assigned less attractive times, no system places any restrictions on total admissions by attending staff physicians or on the days when certain physicians can admit patients or the category of these patients.

In sum, it was our finding that there have been few, if any, really satisfactory scientific methods developed for regulating the size and composition of a medical staff. To date, hospitals have been largely unwilling to devise restrictions for reasons of growth, quality, and legality. Without these types of controls, however, hospitals run the risk, both collectively and individually, of putting unacceptable pressures on the facilities they have available.

It seems to us that restrictions on admissions may well become the reality for hospitals in a highly regulated environment. With per diem reimbursements tightly controlled and the ability to add or eliminate beds and services severely limited, hospitals cannot admit an unlimited number of physicians without injuring patients, doctors, and other hospitals. In many respects, it is unfair to ask the individual institution to face what is essentially an industry-wide problem. Thus guidance from the AMA, the AHA, or appropriate governmental bodies would seem to be in order.

VIII

Conclusion

The complexity and length of this report reflects the wealth and diversity of information that we were able to gather in our brief study of fifteen hospitals. Chapter I of the book was intended both to describe the objectives of the study and to summarize our major conclusions. To repeat these conclusions here seems unnecessary.

Instead, we would like to end the report by offering the reader a list of questions, related to our major conclusions, which emerged during the course of our study. This list proved to be of substantial value in organizing what we learned at the individual hospitals and in evaluating our own institution and its needs. We believe that these questions can be of value as an analytical tool for other institutions as well. Each of the questions must, of course, be considered in light of the specific circumstances of the individual hospital. Thus, certain questions may have to be modified to some degree.

1. MAXIMIZING PHYSICAL CAPACITY

A. What is the hospital's normal and peak inpatient capacity?

   What factors are taken into account (and how) in arriving at the latter number?

B. How many temporary beds are in use during periods of maximum demand?

   Where are they located?

How does the hospital assure itself that the patient will receive medical care that is equal to or better than the care that would be received in a regular bed during the period the patient occupies a temporary bed?

How are patients requiring monitoring handled while in temporary beds?

C. How does the hospital assure itself that outpatient beds (e.g., those supporting one-day surgery or those tests and therapeutic procedures that require a brief period of bed rest by patients) are not considered to be inpatient beds for licensing purposes?

D. Does the hospital have a holding area for patients waiting to be picked up after the established discharge hour?

E. How does the hospital maximize the use of its physical capacity? For example:

Do the size and physical arrangement of nursing units, emergency room, operating room suites, etc., facilitate rather than impede maximum (normal and peak) use?

Do the physical arrangements and medical practices permit reasonable flexibility in the use of beds for different diagnoses or, by their rigidity, effectively make the hospital an agglomeration of sub-hospitals?

Is the basic approach to establishing safety factors for after-hours emergency admissions realistic in terms of the hospital's own experience, the alternatives available in neighboring hospitals, and statistical probability?

Have neighboring hospitals established cooperative, interinstitutional arrangements for handling peak demands? What are they? Has there been adequate medical-staff participation and support?

Is the physical capacity of key hospital departments, particularly operating rooms, sufficient to prevent their becoming limiting factors on the hospital's ability to make full use of available beds?

2. Maximizing the Use of Beds through Policies and Practices of Admitting and Scheduling

A. Does the hospital and its medical staff have a set of overall policies and strategies with which its admitting and scheduling policies and practices are in harmony? How has it reconciled such frequently conflicting objectives and factors as:

— the pressure for beds caused by chronically high occupancy
— the desire to serve the doctors on its staff and their patients as fully as possible
— the medical requirements of particular patients, especially of longer-stay patients
— the desire to minimize fluctuations in the hospital census in the face of, among other things, a short length of stay
— the limitations on service capability imposed by the work schedules of those providing hospital-based medical and surgical services
— patient and community reactions
— financial consequences

B. Given the uncertainty of demand, what buffers and buffering techniques are most heavily in use, for example:

— the cancellation (postponement) of elective admissions
— the acceleration of discharges
— the referral of patients to other doctors and/or institutions
— less convenient solutions, for example:
  1. the more extensive mixing of diagnoses
  2. the use of temporary beds
  3. A.M. admissions, "blind" admissions (admitting surgical patients without a specific room assignment), and other techniques shortening the period between admission and operation

— increased off-peak use

How effectively do these and other techniques cope with the problem? Why?

How does the hospital decide how to use the whole battery of techniques in a balanced approach? Who makes this decision?

C. What priority system is in effect when the hospital cannot handle all patients desiring or requiring admission? What consideration, if any, is given to persons who have previously been cancelled, patients whose PAT work will become outdated by delay, date of reservation, impact on individual doctors, etc.? How are patients' individual needs evaluated?

D. To what extent does the medical staff participate in and support present admission and discharge policies and practices? What steps are taken to prevent abuses in high-occupancy situations?

E. To what extent are admissions and operating room schedules integrated and balanced? How, and how effectively, is this accomplished?

F. To what extent, and how are admissions related to the needs for beds in the upcoming five- to seven-day period and the anticipated availability of those beds rather than simply the need and availability on the day of admission? For example:

> Are elective admissions scheduled to make optimal use of days when occupancy levels are traditionally lower (i.e., is the postoperative recovery period planned to include the weekend)?

> Are elective admissions to specialized nursing units (such as ophthalmology) scheduled to balance the workload throughout the week?

G. Are efforts made to employ the stretchers or beds in the one-day surgery unit more than once on a given day in connection with one-day surgery or diagnostic and therapeutic procedures?

H. How quickly and reliably is information on bed status, patient discharges, transfers, etc., communicated to the admitting office by nursing, housekeeping, and/or patient transport?

> What would be required to improve it?

> How well and cooperatively do the admitting office and nursing units work together on both admission and bed assignment/reassignment problems?

I. How aggressively and in what ways do the admitting office and its policies promote the use of off-peak periods?

J. Are the turnaround times achieved by the housekeeping department in preparing a bed or room for use by a new patient consistent with the needs of the admitting office? What opportunities exist for improvements in performance?

3. PROVIDING HOSPITAL-BASED SERVICES THAT SUPPORT A HIGH RATE OF OCCUPANCY AND A SHORT LENGTH OF STAY

A. Are those services that are provided by hospital-based departments and hospital-based physicians sufficient (in terms of scope, speed, hours and days of coverage, and classifications of patients served) to facilitate or make feasible a high rate of occupancy and a short length of stay? In particular, what is the situation with respect to the following:

Radiology	Operating rooms
Laboratory services	Physical therapy

B. To what extent are there problems of coverage — hours, scope, and/or class of patients — during nights, Saturdays, Sundays, and holidays?

What is the impact on bed utilization, patient admissions, and patient progress?

Do the problems relate to the reluctance of the hospital to assume the cost of extending services or to the reluctance of the hospital-based physicians to provide expanded coverage?

Do attending physicians really want this expanded coverage? How have they expressed this desire? What is the hospital's experience, present policy, and probable future course of action with respect to making off-peak support services available?

C. How extensively is preadmission testing utilized? For what period are test results considered reliable? What is the basis for deciding which tests must be repeated if an admission is postponed? What expedited procedures, if any, are in use for patients not undergoing PAT as the result of hospital policy, urgency of admission, etc.?

D. How good are test turnaround times? What are the major points of delay that presently exist? What, if anything, is being done to identify and reduce them? What delays have been substantially reduced in the past? How was this accomplished in each of the major areas involved (specimen procurement or patient transport, procedure scheduling, interpretation, dictation and transcription, and the communication of test requests and results)? How do test results get on the chart?

E. What efforts are made to coordinate the availability of test results with doctors' needs and daily work habits?

F. What practices are followed with regard to providing physical therapy on weekends, given the accepted medical opinion that early and continued therapy makes a significant difference in a patient's rate of progress?

G. How extensive is the operating-room service that is available for non-emergency patients during late afternoons, evenings, Saturdays, and Sundays?

Has the hospital considered more extended hours than presently offered? With what rationale and decision? What are the perceived barriers?

H. How does the hospital view future trends in surgery in terms of numbers, hours, and complexity per patient/day?

What has been the hospital's experience with outpatient or one-day surgery?

Has it considered dedicated operating rooms for one-day surgery, "lumps and bumps" rooms, off-campus surgical centers, and other alternatives to the main operating room suite?

What does the hospital believe future developments will be?

I. What efforts have been made to increase the effective capacity of the operating rooms by efficient scheduling and management? How effective have they been?

J. Does the fact that the laboratory and radiology departments provide extensive outpatient services affect an inpatient's progress for better or worse to any significant extent?

If so, has this or the fear that a negative effect might occur, led to a change in policy or practices or the establishment of limits, priorities, etc.? What are they?

K. What is the hospital's policy with respect to the acceptance of the work of external laboratories and radiological services?

What are the effects of and basis for this policy?

L. How quickly can an attending physician expect to obtain a consultation from either a hospital-based physician or a specialist?

What steps would improve this situation?

4. REDUCING THE REQUIREMENTS
FOR BEDS BY THE USE OF NONHOSPITAL FACILITIES

A. Does the hospital reduce bed requirements for the diagnostic aspects of a patient's illness by encouraging preadmission testing?

To what extent does it permit the use of nonhospital facilities for this purpose?

B. Does the hospital provide one-day and outpatient surgical services?

What are the scope and volume of operations performed? What trends (numbers, variety, complexity, and risk) are anticipated?

Are dedicated facilities now used or contemplated?

C. What other attempts are made to treat potential inpatients as out-patients in the well-equipped doctor's office or at home?

How successful are they?

What are the major factors affecting the success failure of those efforts?

Have significant attempts been made to influence community attitudes in this regard? With what effect?

D. Which of the following essentially posthospital care facilities are used by the hospital's doctors and patients:

— nursing homes and extended care facilities
— home care, visiting nurses, homemaker, "meals-on-wheels"
— rehabilitation programs, centers or hospitals
— hospices
— mental health centers
— support organizations like Alcoholics Anonymous

What are the attitudes of patients, doctors, and hospital toward their use? Which affiliations have proven particularly effective? What improvements are needed?

E. If well-developed alternatives to hospital care are not available in the community, does the hospital have a program to assist in developing or strengthening them or of developing and operating such agencies itself? If good alternatives exist, has the hospital developed a satisfactory or preferred position with the agencies as the result of its support of and coordination with their efforts?

What is the nature of this support and coordination? Where the reimbursement system does not adequately support the coordinated use of alternative care facilities, what efforts are made by the hospital to alter the situation?

F. Does effective discharge planning exist?

Does it start soon enough — before admission, if need be?

Does it have good communications with patients, doctors, nurses and external agencies?

G. What role do preventive medicine, public education, screening, and physical examinations and the like play in the hospital's efforts?

5. MINIMIZING HOSPITAL STAYS

A. What is the hospital's length of stay — in total, for the major clinical services and for selected, indicative, major diagnoses? Internally, how do these figures compare with historical trends? How do they compare for the region and for other outstanding hospitals? What are the major reasons for the differences (to the extent they are known or can be speculated about)?

B. What kinds of future trends in length of stay does the hospital anticipate? What are the key determinants?

C. If, for some internal or external reason, the hospital had no choice but to reduce its overall length of stay by one-half, one or two days what would it consider to be the most productive areas and approaches?

D. Do the patients, the doctors, and the hospital staff have an understanding of the importance and implications of short patient stays? Do they have a knowledge of what "short" is in sufficient detail and for a sufficiently broad number of diagnoses to develop reasonable goals and expectations? Are the right people providing the necessary information in the right format? Is there proper community preparation or acculturization for short length of stay?

E. Is there an effective utilization review/medical audit function? Are the standards realistic in terms of the achievements of other outstanding hospitals or unrealistically easy in their goals? Are efforts focused on identifying and curing problems — problem areas, problem diagnoses, problem doctors — as well as preventing abuses? Is effective use made of concurrent (by contrast with retroactive) audit procedures? Is the process backed by informative statistical data? Do the utilization and medical audit functions have strong leadership and respected talent throughout? Are these backed strongly by the interest and support of the medical staff and trustees? Do these functions produce results and changes where they are in order?

6. Developing Constructive Managerial, Medical-staff, and Community Attitudes about Length of Stay and Related Matters

A. Do trustees, medical staff and administration all contribute in an appropriate manner to the formulation of policies, strategies, and operating practices? Are channels of communication open in both directions so that problems and potential improvements rise to the surface?

B. Are the board, medical staff, and administration sufficiently aware of the forces at work in the hospital's political, regulatory, fiscal, and social environments? Do they understand both the general trends and the possible major impacts of regulatory mechanisms such as bed complement controls, length of stay controls, reimbursement limitations and denials, PSRO controls, and the like? Of the pressures of business, unions, and commercial insurers on Blue Cross rates, the influence of HMO's and IPA's proprietary hospitals, etc.? Are the risk-reduction opportunities of "running a tight ship" appreciated?

C. Are there adequate efforts to acquaint the general community from which patients originate and the administrative, medical, and nursing staffs of the hospital with the benefits and objectives of short lengths of stay? Are they aware of what this means in sufficiently concrete terms to form a set of reasonable expectations as to how long average patients may expect to stay?

D. Does the hospital use the various resources available to it to influence legislative, regulatory, and community attitudes in such a manner as to promote and reward efficient and effective hospital operations? In what respects and by what means is it most successful in accomplishing this objective?

E. Does the hospital recognize that optimal overall results may best be achieved under policies and practices that submaximize (i.e., operate at less than maximum efficiency) some of the individual units? Which are the major departments that are affected? How is the balance struck?

F. Do admission policies of the medical staff attempt to balance the influx of new doctors with institutional bed availability? What criteria are utilized for selecting physicians and what relative weights are attached to them?

- need to strengthen existing specialties
- need to add new specialties or subspecialties
- candidate's age and existing age distribution
- training and experience
- communications skills
- patient service area, office location, identification with the community
- research competence and experience

Appendixes

APPENDIX 1

A BRIEF DESCRIPTION OF THE VALLEY HOSPITAL

Valley is a 387-bed community hospital, located in Ridgewood, New Jersey, sixteen miles northwest of the George Washington Bridge entry to New York City. It is the primary hospital for the seventeen towns and 225,000 people in its service area, with 19,646 annual admissions (including 2,500 one-day stays).

The percentage of population served by Valley varies from over 95 percent in towns located close to the hospital to about 35 percent in towns located at the periphery of its area. About 35 percent of the patient days are paid under Medicare; less than 5 percent are paid by Medicaid or county welfare programs or provided without charge. Valley's beds are allocated as follows: (273 medical/surgical, 16 CCU, 12 ICU, 43 OB / GYN, 23 pediatrics, and 20 psychiatry). Valley has eight operating rooms. It has a well-equipped laboratory, and an x-ray department with a Computerized Tomography (CT) body scanner, ultrasound, two gamma cameras and a 4 MEV linear accelerator for radiation therapy. It carries out complex diagnostic and surgical procedures (e.g., cardiac catheterization, artificial joint replacements, and neurosurgery) but does not undertake open-heart surgery, organ transplants or Level III perinatology.

In 1979, Valley's length of stay was 6.0 days, as computed under New Jersey regulations, which include one-day-stay surgical patients in inpatient totals. With one-day-stay surgical patients excluded from the inpatient count, Valley's LOS would have been nearly 7.0 days.

APPENDIX 2

A CASE STUDY:
"GETTING THE MOST OUT OF THE HOSPITAL"

Dr. M, a general surgeon, was interviewed one afternoon at about 3:00 P.M. During the interview, he commented on a patient (Mr. F) who had just been hospitalized, with a tentative diagnosis of cancer in the lower gastrointestinal tract. He did not believe it was an emergency. However, he thought it was important to rapidly proceed with the care of the patient. He had ordered a barium enema and asked it to be done *that evening.* At about 3:45 P.M. Dr. M answered a phone call from a pediatrician who had a five-year-old girl in her office with a severe abdominal problem. The pediatrician and Dr. M agreed that the little girl should be hospitalized. Dr. M advised the pediatrician to admit the patient and to order lab work and a flat plate of the abdomen. His discussion of the process, particularly at this time (nearly 4 P.M.), is interesting. He said: "One of the problems is when she presents herself...to the Admitting Office... they have no way of knowing whether [or not] this is an elective case. It's written here 'abdominal pain,' but they don't know if she has had an abdominal pain for two years [and] is going to be worked up, or what. So it's possible that she will be asked to sit in the waiting room while they take three or four people since this is their busy admitting time. This is when tomorrow's surgical [cases] are coming in. . . . Once she gets on the floor, I would think we'd have it all [lab work and x-rays] in an hour. I must admit that personal contact and personal pushing from [me]...will help and I am not beneath taking the person myself in the wheelchair over to x-ray and get x-rays taken. I mean, if you let things go the usual routine way, people working in the hospital don't know how urgent it is. They have no way of knowing. . . . So where I get into the act is letting the people know that this is urgent. They should get the x-ray now. The only way I know to do this is to tell them myself, you know. . . not demanding, not nasty. . . just say, 'This little girl's got a problem, we might be operating on her. Would you get her as soon as you can.' Usually they respond."

The important thing about this quote is that this is what Dr. M said *before* he got up from the chair and said, "Let's go over to the hospital and see what happened." We drove over, walked into the x-ray department and found the child on the x-ray table. The x-ray had been taken. Dr. M felt the child's abdomen and made a tentative diagnosis. He then viewed the flat plates of the abdomen of the child with the radiologist who was in attendance. The discussion with the radiologist did, in fact, somewhat change Dr. M's diagnosis. He commented that it was important and valuable to him that the radiologists were available until 8 P.M. on a regular basis.

Dr. M then discussed Mr. F (an elderly patient, about 70 years old) with the radiologist and asked him to perform the barium enema that evening. We proceeded upstairs to see Mr. F. Dr. M examined the patient's abdomen and then wrote some orders on his chart. Next we went to pediatrics. An IV had already been started on the child and the telephoned report of the laboratory work ordered by the pediatrician was on top of the chart. Based on his reexamination of the child, the laboratory report, and the previously discussed x-ray examination and report, Dr. M decided to take a conservative approach and wait until the next morning for further action. Dr. M then had dinner with the pediatrician in the cafeteria where both of them agreed that this was an appropriate course to follow.

After dinner Dr. M checked on the progress of the barium enema for Mr. F. He found that the patient had not yet been prepared for the barium enema because an EKG technician had come to take his EKG. Dr. M pointed out that one of his options was to have indicated the order in which the various procedures should take place — to give first priority to the preparation for and completion of the barium enema in advance of or in place of other procedures. He acknowledged that he had failed to do this. As such, he did not have the barium enema results yet. This was at about 5:30 P.M. Nevertheless, the patient was now being prepared and was expected to have the barium enema that evening. It was clear that this was not an unusual occurrence in this hospital's radiology department. No one seemed to be disturbed about it. It required little discussion and no apology or pleading from Dr. M.

The message in this vignette is that the doctor knew the system and how to make it work for him in handling two patients promptly and in rapid sequence. His personal attitude and friendliness with hospital personnel and his obvious devotion to his patients' problems were important also. Hospital personnel were neither surprised nor aggravated by his behavior. That Dr. M expected the child to be admitted quickly, taken to the laboratory to have her tests done, and the results phoned to pediatrics and placed on top of the patient's chart, were accepted as routine. That the radiologist was there to discuss a case with the attending surgeon and to do a nonurgent barium enema in the evening was accepted as a matter of course by Dr. M.

Selected Bibliography

Coffey, Richard J. "Preadmission Testing of Hospitalized Surgical Patients and its Relationship to Length of Stay." Ph.D. dissertation, The University of Michigan, 1975.

Commission on Professional and Hospital Activities. *Length of Stay in PAS Hospitals by Diagnosis, Western Region, 1976.* Ann Arbor, Mich.: 1977.

Davidson, Sharon Van Sell. "Components and Systems for Utilization Review." In *PSRO Utilization and Audit in Patient Care*, Sharon Van Sell Davidson, ed. St. Louis: C.V. Mosby Co., 1976.

Frobese, Alfred S. "A Surgeon's View of Ambulatory Surgery." In *Ambulatory Surgical Centers*, Thomas R. Donovan, ed. Germantown, Md.: Aspen Systems Corp., 1976.

Goldberg, George A. and Holloway, Don C. "Emphasizing 'Level of Care' over 'Length of Stay' in Hospital Utilization Review." *Medical Care*, 13, no. 6 (June 1975): 474–485.

Griffith, John R.; Hancock, Walton M. and Munson, Fred C. *Cost Control in Hospitals.* Ann Arbor, Mich.: Health Administration Press, 1976.

Hamilton, Richard A. "The Relationship Between the Timeliness of Diagnostic Test Results and Length of Stay Patterns." Ph.D. dissertation, The University of Michigan, 1979.

Holloway, Don C. and Holton, John. "Mechanism for Evaluation of a Utilization and Audit System." In *PSRO Utilization and Audit in Patient Care*, Sharon Van Sell Davidson, ed. St. Louis: C.V. Mosby Co., 1976.

Holloway, Don C.; Holton, John P.; Goldberg, George A.; and Restuccia, Joseph D. "Development of Hospital Levels of Care Criteria." *Health Care Management Review*, 1, no. 3 (Summer 1976): 61–72.

Holloway, Don C.; Restuccia, Joseph D.; Sondik, Edward; and Kuskey, Kenneth. "Level of Care Decisions by PSROs for Health Facility Planning." Paper presented at the conference/workshop on National Health Policy Issues, sponsored by the Office of Planning, Evaluation, and Legislation, Health Resources Administration, DHEW; San Francisco, California; February 12–13, 1976.

Hospital Utilization Project. *HUP Length of Stay: 1977–1978, Mid-Atlantic Region.* Pittsburg, Penn.: 1979.

Magerlein, David B. "Maximum Average Occupancy and the Resultant Bedsize of Inpatient Hospital Units." Ph.D. dissertation, The University of Michigan, 1978.

Magerlein, James M. "Surgical Scheduling and Admissions Control." Ph.D. dissertation, The University of Michigan, 1978.

Magerlein, James M. and Martin, James B. "Surgical Demand Scheduling: A Review." *Health Services Research*, 13 (1978): 418–433.

McDonnell Douglas Corp. *California Length of Stay, 1977*. Hazelwood, Miss.: 1978.

Perry, Ronald F. "A Simulation-Based Planning Model for a Radiology Department." Ph.D. dissertation, The University of Michigan, 1974.

Perry, Ronald F. and Baum, Richard F., "Resource Allocation and Scheduling for a Radiology Department." In *Cost Control in Hospitals*, John R. Griffith, et al., eds. Ann Arbor, Mich.: Health Administration Press, 1976.

Restuccia, Joseph D. and Holloway, Don C. "Barriers to Appropriate Utilization of an Acute Facility." *Medical Care*, 14, no. 7 (1976).

Scher, Zeke. *The Denver Connection*. Englewood, Colo.: Estes Park Institute, 1976.

Stimson, David H. and Stimson, Ruth H. *Operations Research in Hospitals: Diagnosis and Prognosis*. Chicago: Hospital Research and Educational Trust, 1972.

INDEX

Admitting strategies, 12, 29–33, 122–23, 124; Morning (AM) Admissions, 15, 34–35, 123; Cancellations of, 30, 34, 60, 123; Layoff or Cooperative Arrangements, 18–21; Room Assignments, 34–36; and surgical scheduling, 65

Ambulatory Care. See Outpatient services

Ambulatory Surgery. See Surgery, Same Day

Alcoholics Anonymous, 107, 127

Alcoholism Treatment Programs, 97, 100, 107

American Hospital Association (AHA) 9, 82n, 120

American Medical Association (AMA) 9, 120

Ancillary Services, impact on total hospital operations, 5, 7, 41–42, 125–126. See also: Consultant Services; Laboratory Services; Operating Room; Outpatient services; Patients, transport of; Physical therapy; Preadmission testing (PAT); Radiology services

Anesthesiologists, 73

Beds, improving availability of, 1, 3, 12–21, 27, 85, 121, 133; temporary, 6, 12–13, 121, 122, 123. See also: Holding areas

Blue Cross, 40, 89n, 107, 129

Board of Trustees. See Trustees, board of

California Length of Stay, 1977 (McDonnell), 85n

Cancellations. See Admissions, cancellations of

Capacity stretching. See Beds, availability of

Cardiac Care Unit (CCU), 13, 16, 17, 31, 57

Commission on Professional and Hospital Activities, Length of Stay in PAS Hospitals by Diagnosis, Western Region, 1976, 85n

Community health care systems, 36, 95–109, 114, 127

Computers, 80–81

Consultation services, Physicians, 73–74, 126

Cost Containment in Hospitals (Griffith, Hancock, Munson), 76

Cost of care, 1, 9, 42

Dedicated minor surgical facilities, 64, 68–70, 126, 127

Denver Connection, The, (Scher), 19n

Diagnosis, variations in length of stay by, 5–6, 42, 48, 82–85; importance of prompt, 91

Discharge holding areas, 12, 15–16

Discharge planning, 12, 37–40, 105, 114, 123

Early day testing (EDT), 60, 62. *See also* Preadmission testing

Emergency medical services system, 14

Emergency room, holding areas, 13–14, 32, 57, 97, 122

Emergency room physicians, role in allocating scarce beds, 32

Extended care facilities. *See* Nursing homes

Family planning, 98

Frobese, Alfred S., "A Surgeon's View of Ambulatory Surgery," in *Ambulatory Surgical Centers*, ed., Thomas R. Donovan, 28n

Griffith, Hancock, Munson, *Cost Containment in Hospitals*, 76

Health education, 8, 96, 97, 128; Preventive Programs and Public Education, 97–104

Health Information Program (HIP), 100

Health Maintenance Organizations (HMOs), 8, 9, 85, 89, 104, 105, 108–09, 129

Health Systems Agencies (HSAs), 2, 75, 86, 106, 114

Holding areas, 12, 13–16, 122

Home Care, 8, 39–40, 96, 98, 105, 115, 127; home health aides, 38; homemakers, 38, 98, 105, 127

Hospice Programs, 99, 107, 127

Hospital trustees. *See* Trustees, board of

Hospital Utilization Project, *HUP Length of Stay: 1977–1978, Mid Atlantic Region*, 85n

Independent professional associations (IPAs), 108–09, 129

Intensive Care Unit (ICU), 13, 16, 17, 31, 57

Kaiser-Permanente Medical Care Program, 3, 33–34, 40, 85, 96, 118

Laboratory Services, 7, 22, 23–24, 51–58, 97, 105, 124–25, 126; response time for results, 51–53; tests, 92, 125

Length of stay, 1, 2, 4, 5–6, 76–90; effect of ancillary services, 42, 53–54, 56, 57–58, 71; comparisons, 86, 128; effect of medical office buildings, 92–93; effect of medical staff, 73, 75, 91–92, 112; and OR admissions, 62; effect of preadmission testing, 59; variations among hospitals 82–85; and teaching institutions 87; in obstetrical services 86–90; and public opinion, 113–14; at Valley Hospital, 133

Length of Stay in PAS Hospitals by Diagnosis, Western Region, 1976 (Commission on Professional and Hospital Activities), 86n

Licensure/Regulation, 17, 123

"Lump and Bump" surgical facilities, 64, 126

McDonnell Douglas Corporation, *California Length of Stay, 1977*, 85n

Medicaid, 9, 38–39, 78, 106, 133

Medical audit, 7, 77, 79, 80, 81, 128

Medical office buildings, 92–93, 104–05

Medical staff, 1, 3, 4, 5, 18–21, 108–09, 111–13, 129; and admission and discharge policies, 37, 123; effect on length of stay, 76–93; limitation of, 9, 117–20, 130; and off-peak availability, 22–23, 25; and patient management, 109; and utilization review, 79–80; of Valley Hospital, 117–18

Medicare, 78, 133

Mental health, 97, 98, 127

Mixed nursing units, 12, 16–17

Mothering classes, 88, 89–90

Numerical evaluation system for medical staff composition, 118–19

Nursing, 3, 13, 16, 37, 60, 80

Nursing homes, 8, 38–39, 98, 105–06, 115, 127

Obstetrics, 14–15, 16, 88–90
Occupancy (inpatient) rates, 1, 2, 4, 21–23
Off-peak hours service availability, 6, 21–26, 33, 121, 123, 124; and utilization of ancillary services, 23–24, 43–47, 52–53, 54, 64, 68, 70, 125
Operating room, 123, 125–26; availability of, 7, 23, 24, 62–63, 65, 127; dedicated outpatient units, 28, 68–70; and laboratory service availability, 55–56; scheduling 24–25, 66–68, 124, 126; of Valley Hospital, 133
Operations Research in Hospitals: Diagnosis and Prognosis (Stimson), 17n, 28n
Outpatient services, 48, 58–59, 97, 115
Outpatient Surgery. *See* Surgery, same-day; Dedicated minor surgical facilities

Pathologists, 3, 52–53, 55, 73, 91
Patients; attitudes of, 25–26; characteristics of, 4; education of 103–04, 114; transport of, 49, 71–73, 124
Perry and Baum, "Resource Allocation and Scheduling for a Radiology Department," in *Cost Control in Hospitals*, Griffith, et al., 42n, 55
Physical therapy, 7, 24, 71, 124–25
Physicians. *See* Medical staff
Post-Discharge Services, 38–40. *See also* Home care; Hospice programs; Nursing homes
Preadmission testing (PAT), 7, 34, 52, 58, 59–62, 91, 115, 123, 125, 126; and radiology services, 47, 48, 49
Preoperative holding areas. *See* Holding areas
Preventive medicine, 8, 96, 97, 99, 128
Professional Activity Study (PAS), 77, 78, 84
Professional Standards Review Organizations (PSROs), 7, 77, 81–82, 129
Public Opinion — effects on hospital utilization, 113–14

Quality Assurance Program, 80

Radiologists, 3, 73, 91
Radiology Services, 7, 22, 23–24, 42–51, 105, 124–25, 126, 133
Recovery room as a patient holding area, 13, 14–15
Regulation, 1, 17–18, 77, 114–15, 129
Rehabilitation services or units, 38, 98, 106–07, 127
Reimbursement, programs and effects of, 4, 8–9, 38–39, 39–40, 77 114–15, 129
"Resource Allocation and Scheduling for a Radiology Department," in *Cost Control in Hospitals*, Griffith, et al., 42n, 55
Room assignment techniques, 34–36

Scheduling, 123–24, 125; A.M. admissions, 31; and cancellations, 30, 33–34; by computer, 28, 29; emergency admissions, 32; off-peak admissions, 33; for the operating room, 31–33, 64–66; and room assignment, 34–36; and temporary beds, 31; and triage, 31–32
Scher, Zeke, *The Denver Connection*, 19n
Screening programs 103, 128
Specialized nursing units, effects of, on occupancy, 16, 34, 124
Stimson, David H. and Ruth H., *Operations Research in Hospitals: Diagnosis and Prognosis*, 17n, 28n
Stress, 100, 103
"Surgeon's View of Ambulatory Surgery, A," in *Ambulatory Surgical Centers*, ed., Thomas R. Donovan, 28n
Surgery, 6, 16, 31–33; Same-Day, 26–28, 63, 68, 69, 115, 124, 126, 127

Teaching hospitals, 87, 92
TEL-MED, 100–02
Transcription services, 50
Transport. *See* Patients, transport of

Triage, as admissions system, 31–32
Trustees, Board of, 3, 80, 112, 119

Utilization review, 3, 6–7, 31–32, 37,
    57–58, 70–71, 77–82, 86, 92, 112,
    128

Valley Hospital, 1–2, 3, 4, 82, 117–18,
    133
Visiting nurses, 38, 39, 40, 96, 98,
    107, 127
Visiting Nurses Association (VNA), 39,
    105

Weekend Services. *See* Off-peak hours
    service availability
Wellness programs, 100, 103. *See* also
    Health Education

About the Authors

Arthur B. Toan, Jr., retired in 1975 as the partner responsible for the management services division of Price Waterhouse & Co. He is the author of three books and more than 75 published articles in the field of management sciences. Mr. Toan is a graduate of Dartmouth College and served for twelve years as a member of the Board of Trustees of The Valley Hospital. He served for seven of those years as Vice-President of the Board.

John E. Peterson is Executive Vice-President and Director of The Valley Hospital, a position he has held since 1968. Mr. Peterson is a graduate of the University of Minnesota and received an MBA in Hospital Administration from the University of Chicago. He is a fellow in the American College of Hospital Administrators.

David B. Manchester is a graduate of Dickinson College (Carlisle, Penn.) and received an MPH in Hospital Administration from the University of California at Berkeley. Director of Planning at The Valley Hospital from 1974–1979, Mr. Manchester is now Vice President at Palos Community Hospital, Palos Heights, Illinois. He is a member of the American College of Hospital Administrators.

RNIA

BELOW